Schizophrenia: Aspects of Care

Schizophrenia: Aspects of Care

SUE KERR RMN

School of Health Studies,
Homerton College, Cambridge

W

WHURR PUBLISHERS
LONDON AND PHILADELPHIA

British Library Cataloguing in Publication Data

A catalogue record for this book
is available from the British Library.

ISBN 1 86156 273 X

Typeset by Adrian McLaughlin, a@microguides.net
Printed and bound in the UK by Athenæum Press Limited, Gateshead, Tyne & Wear

Contents

Contributors

Joe Frankland was born and brought up in the Fens, and has lived in East Anglia all his life. Current interests include improving the quality of care for people with a diagnosis of schizophrenia, using his experiences to help others survive schizophrenia and move on by accepting and working with their experiences and building on their strengths.

Sally Goldspink works as a senior occupational therapist, specializing in the area of severe and enduring mental illness. Sally works both as a community-based clinician and a professional teaching associate at Homerton College, Cambridge, School of Health Studies. Her interests include social functioning and cognitive disability (an advocate of the Allen Cognitive Disabilities assessment). Sally has close links to and utilizes Thorn principles and practice.

Trevor Jameson has spent over twenty years working in the field of mental health in London and East Anglia. He has worked both in hospital and community teams. He is currently working as a Jungian Analyst in private practice in Suffolk.

Sue Kerr has worked as a mental health practitioner for people with psychosis for twenty years, and the past ten as a Thorn practitioner. She is currently employed as a Mental Health Lecturer and Thorn programme leader at Homerton College, Cambridge, School of Health Studies. She is interested in raising the quality of care given to individuals who suffer from psychosis.

Sarah Newman is a registered mental health nurse and Thorn practitioner (BA Hons). She is currently working as a community Thorn practitioner in Suffolk, with a particular interest in carers and families of sufferers of schizophrenia.

Ronald W. Ryall is a neurophysiologist by profession, with a special research interest in antipsychotic drugs. He is a Fellow of Churchill College, Cambridge, a member of the Mental Health Act Commission and chairman of its Consent to Treatment Group. He was the chairman and co-ordinator of the Cambridge Group of the National Schizophrenia Fellowship for about 15 years and a National Trustee of the NSF for about 8 years. He is currently the chairman of a registered charity, the Cambridge Pringle Group, which he founded to run sheltered accommodation in Cambridge. One of his daughters was diagnosed as schizophrenic in 1976, although this was later changed to a diagnosis of bipolar disorder.

Introduction

Sue Kerr

The history of the care and treatment of individuals suffering from schizophrenia is not a happy one. Despite considerable advances in pharmacological, psychological and social management of the illness, the clinical outlook remains fragmented, even chaotic. Schizophrenia is a highly complex condition, which impacts on every aspect of an individual's well-being. Today many clinicians are involved in any individual programme of care, and there can be conflict between the different professionals about the weighting of the approaches to the management of an individual's experiences, together with a divergent understanding of the psychological and social consequences of these experiences.

The face of psychiatry has changed beyond recognition in the past 50 years. The most notable changes include the discovery of neuroleptic medications, the closure of the large mental institutions and the devolution to community care, and the growth of interest in psychological interventions for psychotic experiences.

Educational programmes for therapeutic clinicians have also evolved during this period, in line with the sociological climate. The focus of care and management of people with schizophrenia now incorporates a range of interventions that need to be utilized in a collaborative manner.

In 1950, at the 1st International Congress of Psychiatry, Manfred Bleuler stated that 'we are in the dangerous position of not understanding each other'. Over 50 years on, we still seem to be in this position. The term 'multidisciplinary' is used to describe the approach of most clinical teams or units. However, there is much empirical and anecdotal evidence that many professionals are ignorant of the knowledge and skills of their colleagues and can therefore be critical of their clinical decisions. This in turn can affect inter-professional relationships. The result is that clinicians may fail to understand schizophrenia in the context of the experiences of individuals and their carers, and people with schizophrenia and their carers in turn may fail to understand the different approaches taken by the clinicians involved in their treatment. This perpetuates Bleuler's 50-year-old realization.

Thankfully we are now able to fill the several hundred blank pages entombed within the cover of *Schizophrenia: New Knowledge* presented in 1957 at the 2nd International Congress. However, Bleuler's accusation remains, as a challenge to the huge amount of research into the understanding of schizophrenia and developments in treatments.

The aim of this book is to bring together different views about working with schizophrenia. The discussions focus on the psychosocial aspects of care, and the book includes personal narratives from a sufferer and a carer as well as contributions from a psychiatrist who practises as a Jungian analyst, occupational therapists and a psychiatric nurse.

CHAPTER ONE

The science of enduring madness

JOE FRANKLAND

> In my beginning is my end.
> T.S. Eliot *Four Quartets* II 'East Coker'

In the autumn of 1988 I wrote this chapter title on a piece of paper, intending to compose a poem. I sat for what seemed like hours with it in front of me, but nothing came to mind. However, I liked the words, particularly the dual meaning of enduring – that something lasts, maybe permanently; and that equally, something must be borne with whatever fortitude an individual can muster.

Of course, writing now in the year 2002 the words have a fresh meaning. Perhaps even those 14 years that have passed have given me an understanding of madness that I would never have been capable of. Why did I use the term 'madness'? I think now, on reflection, that it was a tacit admission that what was happening to me at that moment was in all ways very strange and that it had been strange for many years previously. However, I did not at the time overtly recognize this. The undercurrents in my life were beginning to drag me away from the shore of reality with greater and greater vigour, until at last I could no longer see the coastline. In the words of Stevie Smith, I was not waving but drowning, cast adrift with no lifejacket in an ocean that grew deeper with confusion and eventual terror.

This time was also the period of my greatest creativity, writing many poems and a novel in the space of three months. I thought I was keeping a toehold on the firm aspects of certainty that we all need. In fact, the many words that came to me in these weeks were simply an attempt to prevent a disintegration of my life, which, subconsciously, I knew to be inevitable.

My story is not a particularly remarkable one. Like every tale, it has elements that are common with others. But equally it is entirely unique in its make-up. I write for you as someone who has gone through certain experiences and now, with the benefit of a newly objective standpoint, feels ready to relate them. These are personal, and very intimate views, but if you bear with them I trust that some sense can be made of what I am trying to do.

Personal history

I was born in August 1965, in the Fenland town of Wisbech. My parents were middle class and professional, both schoolteachers; though they had both in differing ways come up from poor backgrounds. My late father, who was 50 at the time of my birth, was orphaned by the age of 9. A rootless, classless man, he was a decent and kind human being whom I loved very dearly, and I believe he loved me back in a very quiet and unspoken way. We were very alike, and I often think of him as I sit and watch the cricket, a passion we shared. Since his death from cancer in 1999 I have thought much about him, particularly how he must have felt about his past, which he spoke little of, with the exception of his army years in the war. He knew that the death of his parents elevated him socially, since the Methodist minister who ran his home saw his potential and educated him via grammar school and university. After college he taught in private schools, and it was in such a role that he met my mother, when they both lodged in Norwich. He could be said to have been completely institutionalized, and was unprepared for the family life that was to become his.

My mother is a complicated woman who at the time of meeting my father was going through a messy divorce. Like me she was born in the Fens, her mother having settled there from Lancashire as a girl owing to her father's ill health. My grandmother married a local man and they had just the one daughter. My grandparents were decent people who worked hard all their lives, though this left them as rather joyless characters. They owned their own house, but my grandfather's occupations – publican, farm labourer and platelayer on the railway – suggest that they were in truth working class. I mention this now because I believe that class has an important role to play in the formation and acceptance of mental illness, and though I can only describe myself as middle class my roots were certainly not so. This insecurity in my background has had much to do with a lifetime's lack of confidence.

My mother is undoubtedly a bright woman who thinks in a conceptual way. She left school at 16 and worked in London during the war as a secretary. No doubt in today's world she could have gone to university and achieved academic success in a simpler way than she eventually did – she finally trained as a teacher and then took a degree with the Open University in the 1970s, followed by a masters and doctorate in the succeeding decade. This came too late to be of much professional use, as she had retired by then, but she continues to write on educational subjects and has been active politically chairing various committees, both locally and nationally. She had a difficult first marriage and the problems she faced during this have affected her in many ways. The one positive thing to come out of it was the birth of my brother, 10 years before me. He himself is a very friendly and affable sort of chap who has carved out an impressive career. He developed epilepsy as a child, but the calming influence of my father, who adopted him when he married my mother, helped him grow out of this. We are quite opposite types – me a thinker, him a doer – though in later years we have become closer, particularly as he has produced a young family in middle life, and I take great pleasure in watching them grow up.

All this seems a very rushed summary of my family and its dynamics, but since space is short I hope it is sufficient to give an idea of where I am coming from. With age I have come to blame those around me less for my problems, taking instead a more objective viewpoint. But since we are all shaped by our environment, it has to be accepted that the influence of family can be very persuasive. What follows is the best recollection I can give of my life to date, and the way it has shaped and constructed my problems. And I firmly believe that the ways I have come to deal with mental illness lie in this past, and how I have come to cope in the present.

1965–1976: The years in the Fens

My story really begins not with my physical birth but, as with everybody, from the earliest points of my recollection. For me it is this, remaining the most significant thing that has ever been said to me. Sometime, when I was probably about 3 or 4 years old, I was told a story by mother. She said that when she was pregnant, she had been thought to be carrying twins. This obviously proved to be incorrect, but a fibroid grew alongside me. The importance of this statement cannot be underestimated, and will be seen to have affected every area of my development. Simply, I felt that somehow I had had a twin brother, that I had lost and myself survived. A lifetime's misconception, maybe, but fundamental to my personality. Half of me was dead – the support I would necessarily have had from this putative sibling was denied me. And with this came the guilt, this feeling of incompleteness, and an unending process of trying to resurrect part of me that had been taken away. It is an enduring and constant theme in my life, and to this day remains with me. Of course, when I was diagnosed many years later as schizophrenic, it took on new meaning. The misconceived notion of a 'split personality' seemed newly resonant.

I was an unhappy child from the first moments I left the family home and went to kindergarten. When I was 2 years old we had moved back to my mother's home town of March, also in the Fens, to live with her parents. It seemed an odd move, because my mother had a very troubled relationship with her parents, particularly her mother. For the next nine years I honestly remember more of my grandparents than of my parents, who were both teaching at the time. What they felt about having a very active small child to look after I was never able to ask. As I have said, they were a rather miserable pair, but given their experiences – they had both survived cancer and lived through two world wars – this was perhaps understandable. I remember a tremendous freedom as a child, for in those days parents seemed to worry less about safety. I ran and later cycled everywhere, and since we had a large orchard, I was a great tree-house builder. But this happiness was not to be continued into school life. From the start I hated education – not because of any academic problems, but because I found it difficult to relate to my peers. Learning came to be a miserable experience, which was both odd and sad for a bright child who wanted to learn. Many years later, when undergoing cognitive therapy, I came to recognize these early experiences, particularly the fear of rejection, as central to the later development of my illness.

So school was to be, and continued to be, a devastating and dehumanizing event for me. It was always thus, and remained with me to the final point of my education. What caused it to be so? Certainly my character as it formed then, dark and introverted, craving affection and approbation from my fellows, was to a large part to blame. I was bright, and I knew it. Intellectually I had no problems with school work, indeed found a lot of it dull and undemanding. I read voraciously, and was schooled fully, to the point of zealousness, by my parents. I still recall my father reading to me every night, not children's books but Shakespeare and the like. By the time I was 6 I had a reading age of 14. No, my problems were not academic. The feeling of incompleteness, of bereavement, that I have already explained, overwhelmed me. Like any lonely child I sought a replacement companionship from my peers. It was not forthcoming. I threatened them with my intellect: they could not damage me in that way. So they did what children do: since they are fundamentally cruel they attacked me at the most vulnerable point in my personality; my need to be liked. They simply did not like me, and made quite sure I knew it. My accent did not help. My mother, who herself speaks well, ensured that I did not pick up the flat, monotone accent of the Fens. It was drummed into me that I should talk properly, in sentences and with what amounted to received pronunciation. It was the bane of my childhood and remained so until much later in life, when I took steps to remodel it. To the other children at school, I seemed stuck-up, a snob. In fact, I was not stuck-up at all. My character, which formed as all do in early childhood, was and is a contradiction. Fundamentally I am shy and reserved, with little social confidence brought about by a lifetime of rejection. But to mask this I am loud and boisterous, quick-tempered and subject to extremes of passion. When I was a child I hated this. All I wanted to do was be anonymous, to fade quietly into the background. But my abilities marked me out; in addition I was quite large and clumsy. I could not help but be noticeable. I felt that I stood out both in the way I spoke and by my physical presence: my seeming ease in the classroom and the fact that I had no problem with exams. I suspect that if I had been someone else, then I would not really have liked me at all.

From the second year of infant school to the third year of primary, I was saved from a total implosion of my very being by a series of excellent teachers, each very different from one another but offering a complementary passage through the years. I continued to be an achiever, but still fundamentally hated the whole process of education. Perhaps it would have been better if I had been taught at home, because I think my parents felt my unhappiness. However, this did not stop their expectations of me, which grew as the years progressed. It was not, however, a completely isolating experience. There were factors in my childhood which were more enjoyable, but because they were working to compensate an essentially depressing and withdrawn child, they did not mitigate the loneliness. I had one really good friend, whom I knew from the age of 2 until I left March at 11 in the summer of 1976. He was a very different character to me, not academically gifted at all and sometimes very moody; but we got on extremely well and played together constantly in these years. He and I built a large tree-house in the orchard behind my home, lifting old wooden sleepers up on a pulley. We were very proud of it. You could see the magnificent church, famous for its roof, from it and hear the bells as they chimed the hours away. On Sunday they rang for an hour: But this always depressed me, as it meant the end of the weekend and the start of another disturbing week at school. I still recall the feeling of sickness this gave me. I sought refuge here among the branches laden with apples. As my time at March came to an end, and I knew the uncertainty of moving was to descend upon me, I experienced what I now see as very early hallucinations; voices that at once comforted but scared me. I was not yet 11.

There are other points to be made about this time in the Fens. The landscape is breathtaking, with its famous big skies, but also very bleak – vast, prairie-like fields extending endlessly to the horizon; also, as I recall, very few trees, except those planted as a windbreak to prevent the wind whipping the peaty soil in dry summers. The communities tend to be isolated, and generally strung out along roads with little behind them; a relic of the times when the Fens were marshes and settlements grew on the islands above the wetlands. A sense of place, of belonging, has always been important to me: to grow up in such surroundings was a telling reflection on my psyche, both introverted and exposed.

So, how best to summarize these first 11 years of my life? Also, to assess my mental state as it stood back then in 1976? My home life, the youngest by 10 years of the six people in the household, and indeed the youngest by 38 years when my brother left for university in 1974, was complicated; dominated by friction between my mother and grandmother and the remoteness of my father and grandfather. My final year of school had been a disaster. I had a teacher who basically disliked me intensely, and for the first time began to stutter academically. I recall my parents coming back from a parents' evening with an ashen look on their faces, as they tried to explain what had been said to them. It was, I think, a great shock. For me it was the first of many subsequent failures; it could be said that from this point in my life I was backpedalling; taking the proverbial one step forward and two steps back. I had always relied on the approbation of teachers to compensate for rejection from my peers. Now even this was to go.

Picture then, this frightened little boy who was innately depressed and socially unable to connect with society. Adults seemed generally to like me, in fact, I think I became a little adult far too soon, and lost out on childhood. But children did not; my equals in terms of age distrusted and bullied me (never physically, because I was strong, but mentally – the cruellest form of torture). I was as backward emotionally as I was advanced intellectually, and developed a fatal need for friendship so close as to suffocate anyone who came near.

I will relate one more set of experiences that may be pertinent to an assessment of a pre-psychotic state. I have always suffered badly from nightmares; until my teenage years I could not sleep with the light off. When I was young I started to see things that outlasted the dream state, lions and tigers at the foot of my bed and such like. Also (and this has only recently changed), the air always seemed blue with static electricity, a picture that took seemingly hours to dissipate. I began to experience an aura behind my eyelids, flashing lights, which I always assumed was a common problem, but I have learned from others it may not be usual.

In retrospect, I certainly began to hear voices by the time I was 10 or 11, though of course I was unable to rationalize this or even realize that it was abnormal. These early hallucinations were generally of what might be described as a benevolent nature, encouraging me to believe I was somehow special. Had my subsequent experiences been different, I believe now they would have developed into delusions of grandeur. Perhaps the literature on psychosis might rubbish these putative theories, but I am only relating, with the benefit of hindsight, what I perceive was happening to me.

Voice-hearing, however, was intrinsically tied into the complicated fantasy world, or rather, so strong and seducing it became, the alternative reality I have always inhabited. I somehow knew that I was different, but considered that what I did was to tell myself stories, complicated scenarios that involved a restructuring of the events in my life into a more positive framework. The key element in this: Outside the reality, I was supported, by my twin, and existed in a place where happiness was not merely the opposite of misery, but something beautiful; a kind of Nirvana. At this stage, and ignorant of any conception of wrongdoing, I felt in control of my thoughts; a feeling that in the ensuing years would evaporate into psychiatric illness.

I leave this period of my life with the memory of it which haunts me still: A confused, already damaged child sitting up in his tree-house, staring across at the church, his head active and alive. He recalled his life to date, the strange concoction of pain and innocence, knowing that this chapter was about to close and another, unknown, one to begin. Already he knew quite tacitly that things could get far worse. He was not to be wrong. As he sat, the recognition that childhood was over flooded around him. A new age was to begin; the age of withdrawal.

1976–1985: The reluctant passage into adulthood

In February of 1976 my parents and I went for a short break in the half-term week. We stayed in a very upmarket hotel, which was a new experience for me. The place was in a beautiful market town. Unbeknownst to us then, six months later it was also to become my home.

After the nondescript architecture of the Fens, it was a joy to be surrounded by fine Georgian houses, and the medieval churches and abbey ruins. My one ruling passion in life has always been the study of the history of architecture; it is a constant factor in my development. So to be in this wonderful place was a revelation. Fine, then, I thought for a visit. But my security has always been in my home, wherever that has been. 1976 was a watershed year, for it was then that home was to be uprooted and moved somewhere new.

The logistics of this move were entirely practical. We needed more money. My mother had been studying for her degree and we depended on my father's income, which was not great. In addition, he was approaching retirement. So she had to get a job, and one became available at a big comprehensive school. She successfully applied for the headship of the department of religious studies. The house in March was duly sold, my grandparents shifted into the almshouses down the road, and in the September of that year we moved to a very small modern house in the centre of town. It was a personal disaster. Coming from a semi-rural existence with acres of space to an urban place with a garden only 40 feet in length was deeply traumatizing. I pulled back into myself entirely. And, of course, there was a new school to be faced. The system of education was different; in March, at 11 and after primary school, everyone went up to the old secondary modern for two years. After this period, the academic pupils transferred to the former grammar school, the remainder continuing where they were. However, in my new home town the middle school system applied, taking children from the ages of 9 to 13. I thus entered my middle school too late, and was taken into the third year.

I have bittersweet memories of this time. The shock of moving took years to dissipate. Even the glorious buildings could not shake me from the perceptions of feeling trapped; as usual I could not relate to people, and developed no real friendships. But in terms of schoolwork I excelled. There have been two periods in my life when existence seemed to be put on hold, and these two years were one of them.

The school was very academic; it was a church-aided institution whose headmaster was a canon at the cathedral. He was only interested in the bright pupils, the rest being left to flounder. The most positive aspect, certainly in regard to my later life, was the girl who was eventually to be my partner.

But it was not enough to prevent my seeping descent into withdrawal. I did my work, got on with day-to-day life but spent more and more time lying on my bed drifting away into the recesses of my mind. Rejection fuelled paranoia, and the feeling that I had had in March that I was special began to be replaced with deep unease, that I was just plain weird.

It was to be fully seven years before I felt secure once again in my home, but by that time my mental well-being was declining quickly. It was worsened inordinately when in 1978 I moved to the upper school – the same one where my mother was teaching. This was one of the worst decisions I ever took, as I was given the opportunity to attend another school, an option then open to the children of teachers. But the other school had a rough reputation, and I did not wish to lose the acquaintances that I had made in my middle-school years.

The four years at upper school were an unmitigated disaster; from the very start, this big institution (1200 pupils) swallowed me up. I felt trapped and isolated again, with all my usual problems of acceptance. Initially, however, things did not go too badly: I carried on achieving good grades and reports.

I have spoken earlier of my clumsiness and size. In the late 1970s I began to put on weight (it has always fluctuated) until I became very fat indeed. This of course made me a target of fun, but it represented more than this. Once again my physical presence was making me stand out and drew attention to me when all I wanted to do was be anonymous. Keeping my head down was not an option. I took steps to remedy this, though, and in a matter of months virtually halved my weight.

Sadly, anonymity did not follow. Nor did the feelings of persecution go away. Paranoia, the earliest of my psychotic problems, began to affect my work. In the fifth form I sat my O levels, achieving good but not exceptional grades, except in English, which has always been my strongest subject although I really have no interest in literature! Then came another huge mistake. Common sense suggested that at Advanced level I should follow the arts, where my skills lay. but my lone friend was a scientist, so I took maths and science so as not to lose his company. I struggled with the work; but this was not the sole reason for my trouble.

In all honesty I can see now that the withdrawal that I used to get through life really began to draw me away from reality entirely. From the time I left

March, life events meant that the voices I experienced became less and less benevolent and began to turn on me. My mind felt more and more over-active, and it became a place where retreating grew less comfortable. Once I had been able to turn these hallucinations on and off, not allowing them to intrude into the realms of real existence. Now this became harder.

1982 was to be the defining point in my illness. The factors involved in its creation came together in one horrible event that sent me spiralling down-wards into a dark and terrifying place. An incident, which is still too painful to relate in any detail, took place. It involved humiliation not only by the pupils but the staff as well. I had to leave, my studies incomplete; this pushed me into my first, and total, breakdown. For seven weeks I would not come out from my room. I remember lying there and wanting to be dead, yet still feel-ing the terror of death that I have always had. I was damned on both counts.

At this point, the content of the voices I heard became set into the pattern they have always subsequently followed. My cognitions then were of total fail-ure, mutilated still further by a feeling that somehow this was all of my own doing. People hated me – that was evident and not merely a paranoid delu-sion. Thus I must be a bad person – a really bad person. In fact I thought I was evil, that the devil had claimed me and controlled me. These may be delusions to an outsider, but to the sufferer they are very real.

There then followed the second period in my life when it seemed every-thing stood still. I had my education to complete, and I could not go back to my old school. Eventually it was decided that I would attend a local public school. This involved dropping down a year, and from being always amongst the youngest in my group, I became practically the oldest. This pattern of pushing things further back and back became constant, as will be seen.

I was terrified by the prospect of a new school and new classmates. Throughout the remains of that summer I became genuinely terrified and unsure as to what lay ahead for me. The terms were shorter and the holidays longer, common at boarding schools (though I was to attend as a day boy).

The headmaster was extremely good, a decent man. I remember the inter-view with him, in his beautiful study – the school was housed in an old country mansion, set in 450 acres of parkland. He did not question why I had left the upper school and persuaded me that the arts were what I should fol-low, along with mathematics. But by the start of term I was in turmoil. On the first bus ride out I felt completely alone.

But luckily there was one boy there whom I had known at middle school, and he was very kind to me, showing me around. He was largely doing the same subjects so we were together a lot of the time. My initial fears were largely unfounded. The beauty of the surroundings and a genuine feeling of pastoral care brought me out of myself somewhat. I threw myself into every-thing very wholeheartedly, taking part in drama and sport, which I had never done before. We had lessons on a Saturday morning, followed in the afternoon by competitive games at home or away with other schools. I had never been so active, nor was to be again.

But there were still the old horrors. Experience had taught me to be extremely wary of any group of students. By the end of my two-year spell there, the familiar taunts had begun. I left just in time.

I achieved well at A level, obtaining a B and three A grades, in addition to two scholarship exams. Attendance at Oxbridge was thus considered a natural step. I applied to Cambridge to read English, though my real desire was to study architecture. In those days entry to Cambridge was usually through the entrance examination. I chose not to go back to school to study for this, instead receiving private tuition. The exams came and went, and though I did not gain entry to my first choice college, largely because of my terrible performance at interview, I was taken into my second choice. I had no real knowledge of this college, finding out at interview that it was a new institution on the edge of Cambridge and not part of the nucleus of ancient foundations. Even at the interview I found it a depressing place, However, this was to be the place I assumed I would spend the next three years. Of course (having been accepted in the January of 1985) this meant I had a period of nine months before going up. I worked in a local restaurant, and indeed continued to do so on and off until 1989. This had disadvantages. As I was no longer physically active, my weight began to increase again. And the hours were difficult – often I didn't get home until 3 am. It disturbed my sleep and encouraged me to spend the following day on my bed. I now had an excuse to withdraw, probably for the first time. In the summer the first reading list arrived. It had 1400 books on it. I panicked; I knew my heart was not in this. Eventually October arrived, and finally the time came to go up to Cambridge. Remember that in actuality I had dropped a further year; my fellows at upper school were entering their third year at university as I entered my first year. This might seem a minor point, but psychologically it was very important. I felt that things were slipping by; that I was losing my grip on the mechanics of education; and since life is so tied up with this process, on life itself.

Up to this point the logistics of studying had kept a toehold for me in the real world. But I was still acting as I had for the past 20 years, drifting away into my head. People assumed I was just a dreamer; and this was exacerbated by parents who somehow thought it was normal for a 20-year-old to spend all his time locked away in his room doing nothing. Warning bells should have been ringing. They were not. My life-experiences had given me overpowering delusions of persecution. But for the next seven years, I still considered that the voices were telling me stories; and that I had some control over them. This was all right in a state of solitude, but the voices became very invasive in public situations. In fact, the slow descent into psychotic illness was about to quicken.

1985–1990: Freefall

My career at Cambridge began as it does for everyone, with matriculation, the process whereby an individual begins the undergraduate years. A group photograph is always taken on this occasion: I can be seen near the front of mine, short-haired and overweight. Life at the university is unbelievably privileged; formal dinners, college servants and the bedders, who clean each room daily and change the bedding every week. But, in my modern college, the rooms were very small, containing only a bed, a shelf, a wardrobe and a desk. Later they were all provided with a sink: initially washing took place in the communal bathroom (serving eight rooms). There was also a kitchen, though most people chose to eat in hall.

I hated life in college from the start: The noise, the lack of real privacy and above all the people on my staircase, with whom I could not engage at all. The course was no better – after all, I had no real interest in English, just an ability in it. There were seven of us studying there; it is a subject that is taught collegiately, not in a Faculty. Under-read and miserable, I took a chance and went along to the department of architecture to see if they would offer me the chance to change course: much to my surprise, they agreed. I then made a mistake – refusing to take the place. To be candid, I was very confused. I am not a natural artist, and architecture is a vocation where artistic ability is very important.

In order to escape the problems in college, I returned home every weekend. In fact it would have been much better to have gone to a university too far away to have done this. I did not properly leave home at this point. By the end of term I was totally at sea.

Christmas came and went, and I prepared to return. The day I was due to go back, while packing, I had a total panic attack. I knew I could not be there again. I phoned the department of architecture to see if they would give me a place the following October: in effect, to degrade (a Cambridge process) and begin as a first year undergraduate again. They concurred. I had deferred once again (and, for the third time, dropped down a year). The remainder of the year was spent working in the restaurant – I was never one for foreign travel, and felt no need to find myself, because I was scared of what I might find.

The years from 1986 to 1988 were better, certainly academically. I had to live in college for the first year (this is compulsory) but this time found acceptable acquaintances. My social circle grew to probably the largest it has ever been. I was still odd, but this was almost endearing and to be entirely honest I think people found me strangely interesting. My course went surprisingly well, though I was deeply uncomfortable in the company of so many gifted and artistic people. I compensated by making minutely detailed models, which I was good at, and it was this that earned me good grades.

And yet I still returned home every weekend. Gradually I cut myself off from everyone again. I began to sit in my room, lying on my bed and crying. And withdrawing. It was at this time that I began to realize that what I had hoped, that I would grow out of what I later realized to be psychosis, was not going to happen. By now grossly overweight, I began to finally turn my back on the world. I lost all control over my hallucinations, and continued to do something that I had done from the first year in college – that is, to go walkabout at night. I vividly remember those nights, in the cold with frost on the ground, my head alive and feeling utterly desperate.

In retrospect, this is the point when I began, at the age of 22, to experience command voices. It was a deeply uncomfortable experience; though since at this time they instructed me only to harm myself, it was not dangerous to others. The general hallucinations settled into a pattern – a single, identifiably male voice which I felt to be inside my head. Visual hallucinations began to increase; but still I was unaware of what was going on.

In 1988, entering the final year of my degree, several big changes occurred. Unlike most others, I did not want to return to college, so I sought a suitable house to rent, knowing I could let rooms out to other students. It is here that I must bring in my partner. She took the decision to move over to Cambridge with me, as she was at this time unemployed. The third room I rented to a girl who had shared with me in the second year. This was again to prove ultimately disastrous. The house was unfurnished, so my future partner and I scoured second-hand dealers for suitable pieces.

For the first time, I felt I had really left home; I no longer returned there at weekends, and since we had a car, we were able to get out and about. I entered the creative spell that I have previously mentioned; and along with my course it meant I was incredibly active. But still I went walkabout; still I heard this (by now largely single) voice.

I am still unsure why at this time I should have entered the final, and most cataclysmic, breakdown of my life. Things in fact seemed very promising. Perhaps it was overwork. Perhaps, too, there were physical reasons – having been extremely heavy again, I dieted strictly and lost seven stone in seven months. Whatever the reasons, I became very unwell. Initially it was thought to be a physiological problem; I was tested for everything from Crohn's disease to ME. Nothing was found to be wrong, but I suffered violent migraines and excessive mood swings. I had once again to degrade, drop another year and start my course again in the third year. But I never really did get going again. I had a row with my current partner, and we decided we could not live under the same roof. The other girl who shared with us graduated and went off abroad. She was to become very significant again. I had always been fascinated by her: she was very beautiful and had constant strings of admirers. She seemed to find me equally compelling; in reality, a doomed tragedy was waiting to happen.

The lease on our home was not renewed, so I was left homeless with a houseful of furniture. My partner found a flat with a girlfriend. Term began again, with me still having nowhere to live. Eventually I got somewhere. I then made a huge mistake; I asked this other girl to share with me. She agreed.

That autumn was a very strange time. Suddenly I was alone with a pretty girl whom I had held a torch for from afar for years. I never began my studies again. The night walks got longer and more frequent; then they started in the day. I began to follow people around, latching on to specific ones, learning their routines and observing them from a distance. Life at the house was almost incestuous. It always seemed to be dark, with just an open fire burning in the back room. I had become a spectre in my own existence.

The descent into dereliction began in the December of 1989. I had started drinking heavily in a pub on the other side of town. Initially to this other girl it seemed exciting. But she could not see that I was becoming so far removed from sanity that addiction was inevitable. I drank more and more, made acquaintance with my future drinking buddies, and started spending my time in what could only be described as a squat – an incredibly squalid place that, remarkably, was rented. I became involved with drugs, particularly cannabis (I had experimented with it earlier but to no great degree). One day after a particularly heavy session, I returned home to find this other woman in bed with an old friend. I exploded: I smashed up the entire house. Unsurprisingly, she left. I never stayed in that place again.

So I transferred to the rented squat, picked up casual work, and drank and smoked my way first though all my savings, and eventually the bank's money as well. Ironically it is during this part of my life that I felt happiest (and least psychotic). I think this is because, after a lifetime of expectation, nobody made any demands on me. They accepted me for what I was: the ex-university boy who chose to live with bikers. At this period, at least initially, all hallucinations subsided.

But of course it could not last. It was the summer of 1990, and the recession was just beginning. Work dried up, and I could no longer support my habits. Things became increasingly tense, and I was totally out of control. I got into trouble with the police, and increasingly desperately behaved in ways which could have been fatal. I realized that I would leave the squalor either in a wooden box or in a panda car. So I left, utterly defeated, and returned to my parents with my proverbial tail well and truly between my legs.

1990–1992: Maelstrom

If life had been difficult before, that was nothing compared to what lay ahead in the next eight months. I knew by now, in this traumatic hiatus, that there was something intrinsically wrong with me; but I still did not know what. My partner and I got back together – she got a job in a nearby town and temporarily moved back in with her father. Eventually, in the late spring of 1991, we got a house together. Immediately I returned to old habits, but this time I drank and smoked dope on my own, at home – always a dangerous thing to do. My partner' s job was full time. I was unemployed. I spent all day on my own. We had to sell the car, so I was further trapped. Financially things were desperate. To further complicate things, the landlord of the house we rented tried to sell us the property, even helping to arrange a mortgage. It was damp and had a particularly sinister feel to it, so we pulled out and bought another property just round the corner.

It would be easy to blame cannabis for my psychotic experiences but for the fact that they occurred long before I had even tried it. Certainly I will grant that it does not help: particularly in the fact that it can make the smoker paranoid.

These days were some of the darkest I can ever recall. I drank, not socially but on my own, day after day. When I found a suitable supply of cannabis again, this became my one comfort; but both drink and drugs ate into our very limited finances.

As I have said, we moved after eight months into another house close by our original home. It proved to be a disaster. Having always rented, both separately and together, at least we had the freedom knowing we could always move on if we were unhappy with the property. Buying, of course, removed this freedom. If ever there was a house that I would have left at the earliest opportunity, it was the one we bought.

But the whole affair was doomed. The property was one that had been renovated by a local builder. The price was cheap – this was a time when house prices were tumbling – but we made several major mistakes. The most unfortunate was not seeing that the house was opposite a factory which we quickly found out operated 24 hours a day. For 7½ years the constant noise of sawing (the factory made fitted kitchens) and trucks pulling up, reversing and suchlike, made the whole experience entirely negative.

In the autumn of 1991, before we actually moved, I began to experience delusions of grandeur again. I felt I could see into things others could not, most obviously (and strangely) that we as humans existed in seven dimensions. I grew very excited by this, telling everyone around me. Fuelled by drugs it all seemed to make total sense, but in retrospect I cannot see now how I arrived at these conclusions. My partner, however, unbeknownst to me at the time, began to draw her own, very prophetic conclusions.

We had no money at all, so in desperation I did something I have always since regretted. Since I was young I had always collected books, on architectural history and theory. I had by this time amassed quite a collection, including some quite valuable volumes. Desperate for some cash, I sold the majority of them, for probably only a fifth of what I had paid. It was an entirely destructive experience. They had been a means of escape; now that channel was closed to me.

We finally moved in the February of 1992. The new house had no heating, only a coal fire in the living room, so we shivered through what remained of the winter. I can still clearly remember the ice forming on the inside of the bathroom window, its patterns reminding me of life at March where we also had no real heating.

There was little time now for me, I realized; things were slipping away at breakneck pace. My partner, now extremely concerned at what I was saying, urged me to visit the doctor. At first I refused, but my mood was swinging to despair and I needed some confirmation of what was going on. So reluctantly I agreed.

I must say now that in fact I had an excellent GP, a caring man who was extremely fair and gave me a lot of time. At the initial meeting (in April 1992) he straightaway put me on a course of antidepressants. But, as he later confided in me, he was certain what the real problem was. The drugs had no effect.

At this stage I was experiencing total voice control. In an effort to stop this, I started banging my head against the wall on the stairs, hitting it again and again until the plaster and laths beneath broke and came away. I just wanted some peace. The voices themselves moved once more into a command state, most notable being an urge to grab the steering wheel when I was out in somebody's car and pull the vehicle off the road. They were extremely hard to ignore. In addition I experienced frightening visual hallucinations, both inside and outside my head. The external experiences were the most terrifying, distortions of the environment and everything around me which I could not rationalize. The scene was set for a final descent.

1992: Diagnosis

On the morning of 10 May 1992 we received a demand in the post for over £500 in poll tax. We had no money. In addition, we had no telephone. I remember the sickness I felt as I walked up to the phone box to telephone my partner at work. I was in tears. Nothing she could say would console me. As I walked home in utter despair, a plan was forming in my mind – or rather, voices were directing me towards a plan.

I purchased a bottle of vodka from the corner shop, and began to drink it and take the antidepressants that I had been prescribed. The vodka disappeared quickly; the voices became more and more insistent. Once again I began to hit my head against the wall, but it offered no relief. Then I was overwhelmed with the most terrible anger. I went into the kitchen and began to pull everything off the walls. Then I dragged the cooker out. It toppled over on to me, constricting my chest. For what seemed like hours I lay under it (it was probably only a couple of minutes). I felt myself drifting out of my own body and looking down upon myself. Unable to breathe, I pushed it off and staggered to the back door, and smashed my head through the plate glass window. For a brief second, I felt a tremendous relief, but then the blood came. It seemed to pour everywhere. I lurched outside, shouting for help and leaning over the garden fence, leaving a pool of blood over our neighbours' yard. But nobody heard and nobody came. By now the pain began, and I realized I needed help. I staggered down to the corner shop and entered. I shall always be grateful to the shop owners there. They had been very friendly and supportive to us in the past. Without much fuss they sat me down, tried to staunch the blood and called for an ambulance. They also called my partner at her workplace.

The ambulance seemed to take an age, but I felt quite calm by now. Eventually it arrived. The paramedics were friendly and non-judgemental; they dressed the head wounds calmly. Mid-way I felt queasy and threw up. Arriving at the hospital I was taken to A&E. Here it all becomes rather hazy. Time seemed to really drag by. I lay on a bed for ages until my head was stitched and plastered and I was given a tetanus shot. My partner and her father then arrived and sat with me looking ashen-faced and pensive. Then eventually the duty psychiatrist arrived and asked me the question I should have been asked years before. Do you hear voices? I could only reply 'yes'. Then came the little tests that are done to establish a patient's grasp on what is going on around them: What day is it? What time is it? Who is the prime minister? Can you count backwards in sevens from 100? This assessment possibly worked against me in the short term. Because I appeared quite rational, it was decided not to admit me then to the psychiatric ward.

The situation was confused by the state of the hospital system at that time. Trust status was being introduced, and fund-holding for surgeries. My surgery was not yet in control of its budget, and sent its psychiatric patients to a large mental hospital nearby. I was given a letter and told to report to this hospital the following morning for assessment. This was to prove disastrous.

We drove back home in silence. My partner tidied the kitchen up as best she could and the man from the corner shop boarded up the shattered window. I knew I could not spend that night in the house, so we decamped to her father's flat. Little was said. Eventually we adjourned to bed, and after a restless night got up with great trepidation for the hospital appointment.

In all this confusion I had gained one thing – or rather one word. Schizophrenia. I was schizophrenic. At last, after 26 years, someone had put a name to the bizarre and often frightening passage my journey though life had increasingly become. The initial feeling was, perhaps strangely, one of relief. But this relief was to prove ultimately very damaging, as will be seen later.

We took the train that Friday morning. My partner had been given compassionate leave, so at least I was not to be on my own. A taxi bus took us to the hospital. Our initial feelings were of dread. It is a vast, Victorian pile, quite grand but utterly institutional. Set back far from the road, approached through a rather forbidding gate with a drive passing extensive gardens, the building has at the front a two-storey block overshadowed by the wards behind it. We reported to reception, handed over the letter from the duty psychiatrist and waited. And waited. The entrance hall was painted maroon, with a rather incongruous gold chandelier hanging down from the ceiling. Time drifted by, over two hours in the end. My partner could not mask her discomfort and concern.

Eventually we were called, and ushered into an office. It was to be the first of many interviews with psychiatrists. This one was a small man who sat behind a huge desk. I felt very insignificant, just one of the many who had no doubt sat there before me. The room was dark and enormously tall: I felt crushed by it. The architect in me winced. The consultant asked what were to become standard questions to me – if I heard voices, were they in my head, or outside? Did I hear a single voice or multiple ones? Did I see things that weren't there? I answered as truthfully as I could. Midway through the interview, the phone rang. The doctor was called away; an emergency on the ward. We were asked to wait outside. After another hour he returned, announcing brusquely that I was in need of medication and would have to be admitted – 'for a minimum of two weeks – quite possibly longer'. A nurse was arranged to take me up to the admission ward.

We were escorted along dark corridors, again painted a dark maroon. I thought back to my college days, and the work we had done on colour theory. Even in my confused state, I knew the walls were of completely the wrong colour – the colour of dried blood, I thought. Climbing a set of stone stairs, we arrived at the ward. It was quite simply disgusting.

The floor was covered with old lino; there was a dining area at the front, a nurses' office and then a lounge. Everywhere reeked of tobacco; old chairs were all around. The patients were dispersed around this depressing environment, scarcely engaging with any of their fellows. A few books and jigsaws occupied a set of decrepit shelves, and there was a miniature snooker table. The washrooms were even worse, dating no doubt from the time of the hospital's Victorian construction – all dark green paint and tiles. The ward was mixed, but obviously men and women were segregated. The actual sleeping took place usually in dormitories of six beds with curtains around, though there were some individual rooms – cells in all but name. The high ceilings which predominated everywhere only added to the depressing feeling.

As we were shown around, shouting and wailing came from one of the single rooms. I felt my life was over. My first contact with other psychiatric patients was entirely distressing.

The nurse tried his best to reassure us: they would be able to help me –
with medication my problems could be eased. But I think he really knew that
this was an awful place where awful things happened. He went off to organ-
ize my admission. I turned to my partner and saw in her eyes what I felt in
my heart. I was mad and ended up where all mad people go: an asylum. We
turned round and left – or rather, ran away.

That Friday night and back home, the hallucinations (for that was what I
knew they were) reached new levels of awfulness.

By the Monday, and feeling desperately ill, I visited the surgery to see my
GP. Unfortunately he was away, so I was passed to another doctor. She told
me what I was experiencing must be awful (little use – I wanted action, not
sympathy) and started me on a course of chlorpromazine. My partner
returned to work and once again I was alone all day.

The drug did nothing for me: in fact the only thing that kept me going at
this time was my community psychiatric nurse (CPN) who had been to see
me before diagnosis. She was a remarkable woman, very strong but friendly.
In addition, my GP began to visit me regularly – quite a remarkable fact given
his workload.

My refusal to be admitted led to an inevitable crisis. I needed help, that I
knew: but I could not countenance going back to the hospital. It was agreed
to see me as an outpatient. So one Wednesday morning my CPN took me
over to the hospital to see my second consultant. After the usual waiting
around, I had about five minutes with her in which she doubled the dose of
chlorpromazine that I was taking. Another incident occurred at this time
which I only found out about later. I was wearing a combat shirt, as I often
did then because they were very cheap. In my notes it was suggested I had a
'paramilitary obsession'! This was deeply upsetting, and an example of the
dangerous practice of judging by appearance. But it was in my notes, and I
had to ask for it to be removed.

Still the drugs did not work. I was back on cannabis this time, which at
least allowed me to retreat once more into my head, though this was now no
longer pleasant. The weeks passed, with no let-up in my symptoms. I visited
the consultant again. She decided that another drug should be tried (always
I felt that they resented the fact that I refused admission). This was to be the
worst incident in drug treatment I have ever experienced. I knew little about
side effects at this time, other than that the chlorpromazine had made me
tired and lethargic.

The drug I was then given was the infamous Depixol (flupentixol
decanoate), administered intramuscularly. I had two doses, each of 40 mg,
on consecutive days. Later I was to learn that this was completely incorrect
practice, and that a dose of only 20 mg should have been given to test my tol-
erance to the drug. For three days nothing happened, but then on the
Monday morning I felt acute back pain. I went to see the GP and was given

paracetamol. By the afternoon my muscles felt acutely active, and I was unable to sit still. This worsened increasingly, until in the end all I could do was just lie on the bed and allow the continuous spasms to occur. Once again I was terrified. What could be done?

My CPN, seeing the situation for what it was – the condition known as akathisia – immediately got me put on a course of the anti-parkinsonian drug procyclidine. But it had no effect – after all, the depot injection of Depixol was designed to last a month. I was out of my mind with worry and fear. The procyclidine had no effect. After five days I was taken over to see another psychiatrist. He seemed more interested in listening to the cricket on his radio than talking to me, but his conclusion was that I would have to wait for the drug to pass out of my system before the restlessness would abate.

Over the following weekend I went out of my mind with worry. It was at this time that many of my later conclusions about medication were made. How could a drug designed to help one condition bring on side effects that were even worse to handle? By Monday I was so desperate that I asked, very reluctantly, that I be taken into hospital. It was a total climb-down on my part, but surely I felt they would be able to do something for me there. Of course I was wrong.

Without a car I had to be taken in by ambulance. My partner came with me, and sat in as the process of admission took place. The nurse who admitted me was built like a prop-forward with arms as thick as most people's legs, but he seemed quite friendly. I was shown to my bed, in the dormitory, and sat on it feeling totally defeated – but of course was still restless and twitching. My partner had to leave about 10 o'clock to catch the last train back home. I remember that feeling of fear and total loneliness as she passed out of the double doors of the ward.

The remains of that evening I tried to spend some time with the other patients. Apart from one, they were all totally unresponsive: but this one chap seemed to want to make a friend of me. We played snooker for a while before retiring to our beds, his being next to mine. I read for a while before finally passing into a troubled sleep.

The following day I quickly learnt the truth: that the akathisia could not be treated. I was already on the maximum dose of procyclidine. I could just as easily take this at home. It was decided that I no longer needed to sleep on the ward, but to monitor me they wanted me there in the day. So I went home that Tuesday evening. The following day I walked from the station to the hospital (some three miles). I was given my pills for the night, and embarked on the long walk back to the train.

At this time it has to be said that my symptoms were quite well controlled; or at least I was so distracted by side effects that I did not notice their presence so much. On my journey I passed a small park, and broke off the walk to rest and have a cigarette. It was midsummer, the sun was hot and somehow I felt I could do things better on my own. I resolved then and there never to take medication again.

Of course this was a mistake; but I was haunted by the experience of akathisia so much that I regarded all medication in the same light – that it would give me terrible physical problems. The resolve was to be sorely tested in the next six months.

The side effects took weeks to subside, but of course as the drugs dropped out of my system, so my symptoms returned. In fact they seemed worse than ever. I could not sleep at night at all, and was haunted constantly by destructive voices and visions that disturbed my very perceptions of reality. In addition, I had not returned to the hospital as I was supposed to, to be monitored. The police were sent round to find out where I was – a deeply humiliating experience.

The six months until February 1993 represent a nadir in my illness. Because I refused all medication, I could not control my symptoms, which worsened with time. Another psychiatrist was sent over and saw me at home in the presence of my GP. He listened attentively for an hour, told me what I already knew – that I was suffering from schizophrenia – and that I needed medication and, preferably, admission. This I refused.

Psychotic events continued to accelerate. I began to have olfactory hallucinations. My use of cannabis increased again, which did me no good. Then, shortly before Christmas, I had a particularly frightening experience which confirmed to me the depth of my problems. I had had a very stressful day, and in the afternoon, after hearing many voices, my partner's father arrived. Quite simply, I refused to believe he was who he claimed to be; I thought he was an impostor. This classic symptom of psychosis seems very strange in retrospect, and I can only explain it this way. Often I have felt that my senses have been heightened, usually at times of pressure. These senses responded to this man and the signals he gave off – he sounded different – were not those I was accustomed to. Therefore it was quite logical to assume he was not who he purported to be.

I was very shaken by this, and it set the tone for a completely awful Christmas. All the usual tools of distraction – music, radio, television – became impossible to use as I was convinced that they were all communicating directly with me – classic ideas of reference. I did not go out much at all, as levels of paranoia had reached impossible proportions. All this gave free rein to my hallucinations, particularly aural: the seed of a persecution complex sown in my childhood blossomed into a state whereby I simply assumed everybody was laughing at me.

This could not go on. After Christmas, and with my partner at her wit's end, I sought help again from my GP. He coaxed me into accepting the need for medication, and without much confidence I reluctantly agreed (to be fair, he did stress that with oral medication it could be stopped quickly if side effects became intolerable). So I started a course of stelazine. It did nothing for me, but I suppose I did not take it for long enough. Life now became unbearable; there was only one thing left to do. I absolutely refused to return to hospital; but that April the GP's practice was to become fund-holding, and intended to purchase their mental health services from another Trust. It was arranged that I would go early as an extra-contractual referral (ECR): so in the February of 1993 I embarked on the second phase of my treatment.

1993–1995: Initial treatment: the highs and lows of psychiatric care

This was a very different institution. To start, the service was provided in a ward in the main hospital. It was a much friendlier place, painted in brighter colours, clean and with a reserved area for smoking, so the whole place did not stink of tobacco.

There were some single rooms, but I was put in a dormitory of eight. There were solid partitions between the beds, rather than curtains, so there was a sense of privacy.

Luckily, for this admission I kept my CPN, though this eventually had to change. And of course there was a new consultant to get to know (my fifth in less than a year). This initial treatment involved putting me on to the relatively new drug sulpiride. It had the effect of calming, if not removing, my overt symptoms. But I was still unhappy in hospital. I was given weekend leave, and felt relieved to be back home. I dreaded Sunday nights, and the return to the ward.

Boredom was the worst factor of psychiatric care, and also the atmosphere on the ward. Most of the time it was quite stable; people very much solitary and non-communicative, but causing no problem. However, a new patient could upset the whole balance of things, for example someone exhibiting disinhibited behaviour. Quickly things would become very tense. Because I was quite articulate still, people tended (and this happened throughout my history of admission) to latch on to me, regarding me as a kind of spokesperson. This felt strange to a man who all his life had experienced rejection and ridicule in social circumstances.

From the outset, however, things did not go well with this new consultant. I scarcely saw him except in ward round. The lasting statement that I remember him saying was very telling. He said to me that people who suffered schizophrenia 'lost their spark' but I had not. So, therefore, though I exhibited all the symptoms of the illness, I had no real problem. It was to be another two years before I trusted a psychiatrist again.

After three weeks I discharged myself (as I was a voluntary patient) and continued treatment as an outpatient. This involved a journey over to the hospital every Wednesday for ward round, an entirely pointless exercise as frequently I was never seen. My CPN had to be changed and I was put with another. I shall always be grateful to the first nurse I had. Her warmth and humanity kept me going through the most trying period in my life.

Back in the community, I continued to take an ever-increasing dose of sulpiride, eventually reaching the maximum of 2400 mg daily. I was also put on carbamazepine, as my consultant was very interested in my family history of epilepsy. In fact he sent me to the neuropsychiatric department of the Royal Maudsley Hospital in London, as he felt I might suffer from temporal lobe epilepsy. This has never been proved either way.

The new CPN was unfortunately unable to visit me at home and so I had to go up to the doctor's surgery once a week to see her. This was frustrating, indeed quite a contradictory state of affairs. The purpose of being treated in the community, I thought, was so you could be seen at home, in the security of familiar surroundings. To have to sit in a busy waiting room while suffering paranoid delusions was not an ideal state of affairs.

This situation continued for a number of months. Once again, though, my symptoms had worsened. In addition I was incredibly tired and lethargic, had become impotent and was starting to put on weight once again. Another, briefer, admission followed. The consultant then thought a change in medication might be appropriate, so I was transferred on to remoxipride, a sulpiride derivative that has since been withdrawn. I question whether any medication would have worked at this time, as my negative cognitions and total lack of self-esteem were as great a handicap as the most florid of hallucinations. I began down the rocky road that is polypharmacy, taking increasingly large doses of various medications for both symptoms and side effects.

The frustration I felt at the weekly ordeal of ward round was finally ended in 1994, when I was transferred to the caseload of another consultant, who visited the GP's surgery once a week and dealt with cases there. At my first appointment with him, I felt immediately that we would not get on, a situation that time proved entirely well founded. This time the new miracle drug was risperidone (it seems strange to me that all consultants seem to have a 'pet' medication). Once again it did little but alleviate the strength of symptoms. About this time my withdrawal from the world had entered its final, complete and total phase. My only exit from the house was this weekly visit to the health centre. The psychiatrist had a very close working relationship with my nurse, who usually sat in on our sessions. Over the months I became increasingly afraid of this, starting to believe that they were conspiring against me. I felt that I was in all ways difficult, readily complaining through frustration at the ineffectiveness of medication. At this time I was also hauled in front of a psychotherapist, to see if some other treatment could be used. He sat and listened very politely to me for an hour, then announced stridently that 'we do not give psychotherapy to schizophrenics as it encourages them in their delusions'. It reminded me of the time when I was first treated, when I was told that I would be ill until my 60s, at which point the symptoms might ease if I was lucky. These two statements still haunt me, a double life sentence with no remission.

I was quite despondent and grew increasingly of the opinion that somehow all this was deserved. Medication was at best a palliative that merely dulled the pain; in addition it made me tired, lethargic and totally uninterested in anything. I still used cannabis to quite an extent now, to escape the awful oppressive nature of the drugs I took (this I know is quite common). Life was very tense at home, though things had improved financially. All the interest I had once had – in sport (I had played cricket and rugby), in music and in architecture – evaporated. My days were spent sleeping, something I found quite easy as the medication was so somnolent.

Even conversation became difficult. And the depression I felt, that had dogged me all my life, began to reach violent proportions. In amongst this were two (half-hearted) suicide attempts, one an overdose and the other the cutting of my wrist. On both occasions it was my articulate defence of these actions which kept me from sectioning and admission. Perhaps herein there lies a dilemma – could it be that my enduring ability to talk my way out of situations ultimately kept me ill for so long? Certainly a lifetime of applied reason was the major factor of my surviving at all, coupled with a total fear of what might lie beyond death.

1994 closed with little improved. Self-esteem worsened – there seemed nowhere to go from this point. But that was before the events of 1995.

1995–1998: Rehabilitation and the long road back

In January 1995 I was finally transferred from acute services to rehabilitation, based in a separate day hospital. The building was and remains a disaster – the architect in me once again still cringes at the Portakabin with a corridor running down the middle and little cell-like rooms opening off it. But the people seemed different. I suppose it is because of the nature of rehab that patients are out of the acute phase of their illness. Here were sown the first conceptions that maybe, just maybe, things could really get better.

So I turned up one January morning to the day hospital, to meet my seventh consultant in 3½ years. He was new to the post, having just taken over rehab services, and took instant action; very decisive. It revolved around the use of the medication clozapine. I remember him saying to me that 2% of patients could not tolerate the drug. I found myself saying – 'well, that means I have a 98% chance of succeeding with it.' It strikes me still that it was one of the most positive things I have ever said.

The use of clozapine on the ward had been, I believe, restricted to only one patient. A 'five strikes and out' rule then applied to its use; that is, a patient had to have tried and failed to respond to at least five other medications before it could be introduced (a condition I easily met). Clozapine and its many derivatives – the so-called atypical medications – have revolutionized psychiatric practice, though my own relationship with it proved to be very stormy and ultimately nearly fatal. However, I am glad to have used this treatment. It opened doors into another world, a world of new possibilities.

After the initial blood tests, clozapine was introduced rapidly and other medications were reduced and finally withdrawn. I still had to take an anticonvulsant, as clozapine increases the chance of seizure. In addition, antidepressants of various type were added in, as the deep underlying sense of depression I felt was still present. But I felt at least some sense of compactness in my treatment, that it was specific to my needs.

The initial effect of clozapine was the reduction of symptoms to a level whereby a sense of normality returned to my mind. The dose was built up, eventually reaching 800 mg a day. I felt I could go somewhere with this: I was marginally less depressed and started to make models and undertake some architectural draughtsmanship again. It is at this point that I must add in my thanks to my partner's father, whose support and friendship have grown to be a very important factor in my life. His acceptance of me has been most positive. I spent much time with him, in the day going up to his flat. We started to go out on Fridays to visit pubs and enjoy a meal and a pint; then visiting second-hand bookshops. This had two important benefits: it provided a degree of socialization, and also re-fired my interest in books.

All seemed to be proceeding quite well. I was still lethargic and by now seriously overweight, and needed a lot of sleep. But there were positive elements growing in my life. My partner noticed the change, and for probably the first time in the duration of our relationship, felt able to relax.

In addition, a good team of nurses and occupational therapists (OTs) was built around me. They were all people I felt I could trust, a complete contrast to my earlier experiences.

But of course fate decrees that life is full of surprises. Mine came in 1996. About the middle of the year, I began to experience pain and stiffness in my joints, particularly those of the lower body. In addition, the hair on my legs began to fall out. What was going on? I broached the subject with my consultant. My blood tests were normal; there was no problem there. Tentatively an idea came to him. He had read somewhere that an extremely rare (several million to one chance) side effect of clozapine was the condition known as systemic lupus erythematosus (SLE), an illness which affects the muscular structures around the joints. It is caused by overproduction of the white blood cells, leading to an over-activity of the immune system which then attacks the body tissue itself. I was sent over for an appointment with the rheumatology department at the hospital. Blood was taken: The results concluded that I did indeed have lupus. It could prove very dangerous indeed, because in an advanced phase organs such as the liver and kidneys could be affected.

But there was also another possibility: could it be that I suffered from lupus regardless of the clozapine; that it was in fact a pre-existing condition (the chances of this, though tiny, were higher than the chance of its being a side effect). There then began a three-year battle between the psychiatrist and rheumatologist as to what to do. The consultant at rehab naturally wanted to continue to prescribe a drug that had obvious therapeutic value; rheumatology on the other hand was aware of the dangers of SLE.

Initially I was put on steroids to treat the muscle pains. Steroids are difficult drugs, effective but quite dangerous, whose reduction must be managed very carefully and slowly. The immediate impact was therapeutically successful but led to enormous weight gain – four stone in four months, leaving me a vast 24 stone. By Christmas of this year I was switched on to other lupus drugs, which simply increased the already rapidly advancing polyphamacy that had, I hoped, become a thing of the past.

The inevitable decision was that I was to cease the clozapine treatment. It seemed most likely that this was the cause of the SLE. Luckily, at this time a new generation of atypical antipsychotic drugs was becoming available. I was tried on sertindole (later withdrawn), which required heart monitoring, then, after much consultation with my partner, asked for it to be reduced to a sub-therapeutic dose. This decision, which may have seemed rash, was taken in the hope that the lethargy and withdrawal which seemed a consequence of all medication (even clozapine) could be lifted, and that I could perhaps once again become creative. It was a short-lived experiment, as my symptoms rapidly returned. (I must add at this time that my use of cannabis finally ceased. Over the years it had proved to be both friend and tormentor.) Also, interestingly, my lupus symptoms gradually began to return. I was put on to the clozapine-related atypical olanzapine, soon at the maximum dose of 20 mg a day. Various antidepressants and also sulpuride were added, and, eventually amisulpride.

In fact, I was increasingly desperate. But there was one thing I had not tried, and that was employment. A friend of the consultant was an architect, and sometime earlier he had been approached regarding possibly using me in some way in his practice – he had agreed. In a last frantic effort to sort myself out, I asked if the offer was still open. It was, and in July 1997 I embarked on a daily train journey to work. It was of course not a proper job. I was not to be paid. But it seemed to give me some self-respect; the partners were friendly and at last I was able to utilize my skills as both a draughtsman and a model maker. I still visited the consultant once a week, walking up from work; but all other contact with nurses and OTs ceased.

For six weeks all proceeded well. I finished a large model and was given a bonus of £100 for my trouble. Then, towards the end of the summer, I broke off for two weeks' holiday. As the end of the break approached, I began to experience voices again and felt acutely depressed. The result was that, when the time came to return to work, I found I could not. This blow was to prove cataclysmic in my life.

The initial reaction was to change medication again, this time on to another new atypical, namely quetiapine. It had little effect; in addition my depression worsened. Also, since all the visits from the nurses and OTs had ceased when I began work it was to prove very difficult for them to timetable me in again. Lonely and confused, I felt utterly suicidal. There then followed one of the worst mistakes I have ever made; to be frank, an error (perhaps not misguided, and certainly his only one) on the part of my psychiatrist. He suggested electroconvulsive therapy (ECT). My partner was at once horrified. It was something she felt innately repugnant and inhuman; that things should have been reduced to this was testimony to the complete awfulness of her – and our – lives. She voiced her feelings but was ignored. Against her wishes and because I had little choice in the matter I agreed: and from that point onwards she will see no one in connection with my treatment.

The actual day of the first session arrived. It was a Tuesday in October. My partner was unable to take me over for treatment, so upset was she; so my mother deputized. I remember nothing of the actual process, except my nerves and the kindness of the ECT nurse; and the migraine afterwards. The second session was on the Friday, also my partner's birthday. Once again I returned with only a severe headache. My partner could only cry; I knew I could do only one thing. I withdrew from the treatment.

So here we were again in a complete mess. The return of the lupus after discontinuing clozapine was taken by the (psychiatric) consultant to mean that it was not the drug that was causing the SLE, so I could return to it. I did, and in a remarkably short space of time was back up to near maximum dose. The polypharmacy increased still further, as I still had to take drugs for the lupus and now to try to cease the hypersalivation that this regime of clozapine had induced.

Throughout the Christmas period, and into the late summer of 1998, my nursing became erratic, largely due to the ill-health of those involved. Clozapine once again was quite effective in treating the positive symptoms of schizophrenia – most notably the hallucinations, particularly aural – but for me its perceived ability to help with the negative symptoms – the lethargy and withdrawal – was negative. My failure at work had completed the demolition of my self-esteem (it had always been a make-or-break choice). But finally something positive was about to happen.

1998–1999 CBT: Better things ahead

In the autumn of 1998, I was given a new CPN from the day hospital, who worked in close conjunction with a senior OT. Immediately the problems I had had with erratic and irregular treatment were nullified. The initial period of talking revealed that in addition to my psychotic symptoms I experienced a high level of anxiety. This was tackled first. It was the primary stage in the process known as cognitive behavioural therapy (CBT) which previous nurses had started but failed to push much further.

It is no exaggeration to say that CBT has changed my life completely. It is not an easy or necessarily quick process; and at the start the still high predominance of my negative symptoms was a handicap. By Christmas the initial work was done. There then came another and eventually beneficial event.

In January 1999 I began to suffer acute kidney pains. I was taken to the rheumatologist who took blood samples and disclosed that my creatinine levels were extremely high – in other words, my kidneys were failing. Her immediate action was to take me off all lupus-related medication; but there was another conclusion to be drawn. This had happened while I was back on clozapine: therefore it was likely that the condition was, in fact, drug related. The psychiatrist had no option but to finally remove the drug from my treatment.

I have always found that the symptoms of schizophrenia become far worse when medication is changed or withdrawn. And this occasion was to be no exception. I experienced terrifying voices and visions, and these were unusual as they were outside my head (in general my voices are heard inside the head) – a whispering in the ear; distorted visions of my surroundings.

Another drug had to be found, and this time it was another atypical, zotepine. This course of medication had no beneficial effect at all, as I experienced severe paranoid delusions of persecution. In fact, it was probably only the sulpiride I was still taking that kept me in any sort of sanity. My anxiety levels were very high and I had to take diazepam to cope with some situations.

But the CBT continued throughout, and gradually I began to cope better. In addition, for the first time in perhaps 17 years I felt real emotion; I began to cry at the slightest provocation. Suddenly part of me that had been buried deep for so long came back: it was at once terrifying and exhilarating. Then, as I still needed a major medication, an experiment was tried, namely the prescription of olanzapine at a very high dose. This was built up to 45 mg a day. For a time the effect was an almost complete abatement of symptoms. A new dawn? It seemed so.

1999–2002: Onwards and upwards

As it slowly became clear to me that for the first time in over 17 years I was no longer cripplingly psychotic, life assumed new dimensions. Now I could go out with no fear of paranoia; could socialize once more and enjoy it; and restart my life. This threw up a contradiction.

Since the age of 16 I had lived in a largely hermetically sealed life. I had ceased to develop. Now, here I was, nearly 34 but with the emotions of a teenager. I was unprepared for the welter of feelings that would engulf me. The mistakes I had made in this period came – and still come – back to haunt me. The two greatest were the social deskilling that had occurred – the loss of relationships, and my failure to complete my architectural training. It must be remembered that I had not worked for a decade; and such a period of unemployment affects anyone, regardless of their mental state. As I said, suddenly to feel emotion again was startling; in fact quite frightening. And another factor that came into play was my depression. I have probably suffered clinical depression all my life, manifesting itself in my failure in relationships and a tremendous fear of rejection.

I liken mental breakdown to passing through a storm. First you enter it, are bombarded with terrifying experiences, and feel there is no hope. When things improve, it is like entering the eye of the hurricane. Everything goes quiet. There is a lull and a feeling of calm, almost elation. But you are not out of it. You must pass again though the winds, battered not by psychosis this time but all the conflicting emotions that have been suppressed for so long.

By this time I felt that I had recovered. But things were not so simple. After the death of my father in 1999, my mood worsened, and the following January I was put on lamotrigine in the hope that it would stabilize this. In fact, as the year progressed, I began to have trouble sleeping, eventually settling at around only 2–3 hours a night. It drove me to distraction, and in desperation I decided to give up all medication. I did this against the advice of everyone, most notably my partner and CPN, and the result was predictable – a return of symptoms, to a level where I became very unwell. I would not speak to my family, and believed in a conspiracy against me. It is true to say that on a positive note I felt much more emotional again, but was so disabled by hallucinations that I was unable to enjoy this. Rapidly I had to climb down and resume drug treatment, but at a much more acceptable dose. Initially I felt defeated and resentful, but as the symptoms receded I came to a kind of understanding of this state we call psychosis. I realize that it will never go away, however much I wish it to – that it will shape and direct my life – but that I can work with it. All the uncertainties remain, but experience tells me I must live with them. We have reached a settlement, schizophrenia and me, and by recognizing this I move forward. This I know now is the closest I will come to recovery – not perfect, not always happy, but quietly stronger.

I know now that I shall never be an architect, or an academic as I had assumed. Initially this was like a bereavement – a sense common in the recovery phase. But through my illness I have gained other skills, above all an understanding of both the cause and effects of schizophrenia. Now I can use this experience; turn something that seemed entirely destructive to more positive ends.

In the September of 1999 I was invited to sit on an interview panel for a programme teaching mental health professional about psychosis. It provides specialist training for healthcare professionals in dealing with severe and enduring mental illness. It was a tremendous boost to my self-esteem, to actually have my views taken seriously and in a small way to shape the future of treatment for people like myself. And since 2000, I have been involved with the actual teaching of the course. It has been most rewarding, and an opportunity to give something back.

During this period, a number of significant life events have occurred. As mentioned, my father sadly died, but we were with him as he passed away and it was a very beautiful, tranquil end. And we have moved house. So I sit here now in a quiet village, enjoying the birdsong, and writing this for you. With all its vicissitudes, twists and turns, schizophrenia is a devious adversary, but I reckon I understand it now. Not a victory, but an honourable draw.

Conclusions: the synthesis of psychosis

At the start of this autobiographical work I asked you, the reader, to bear with it. As a story it is unique; even perhaps if it mirrors some experiences you have dealt with in your professional lives. I hope it gives some understanding of what constitutes the process of mental breakdown, its causes and effects. Now it is time to draw from it the conclusions I have reached. You will not read them in books, or at least most of them. They are personal, and must be treated as such. Perhaps you will not relate to them, or to only a few. But it is a perspective on psychosis, and any perspective in life has a value.

Setting the parameters

First I must say that I am not a patient, or at least not any more. The word 'patient' implies a dependency, usually on professionals: it also implies subservience. A doctor is there to treat you; he or she is the person who knows best and you had better do as the doctor says. There is a theory that the practice of psychiatry is self-fulfilling, in that it simply creates patients so that there is somebody to treat. A means to its own ends. I prefer to be referred to as a client, or service user. This gives me some autonomy and a degree of respect. It also shows that there is a service which I am utilizing, for my own problems and needs.

Second, I am not schizophrenic. As I said in the autobiographical section, when I was first diagnosed I told everyone around me. This was to prove a big mistake: of course they all ran away, their understanding of the word both prejudiced and confused. I am somebody who suffers from schizophrenia, a schizophrenic illness, or (as I prefer) a psychotic disorder. This terminology does not define me as an illness. I am a person first and foremost, whether I am ill or not. These may seem trite points, but if the balance of treatment of psychiatric problems is to change, then it must surely be a move towards encouraging the self-belief of clients. In the end, we can help ourselves perhaps far more than professionals think.

Telling myself stories: a journey through the battlefield of hallucinations

Hallucinations are well documented and factual. They affect all the senses, and I have experienced them in all of the five areas. The most powerful, common and in many ways destructive is the hearing of voices. Received wisdom suggests they can be single or multiple. We all know the bag-lady in the street, shouting at nothing. Usually we cross the road or turn away uncomfortably, trying to pretend she is not there. Voices can be both benevolent and critical: as I have said, in the early stages of my illness, they encouraged me to think I was special, and had knowledge that others could not share. Even as late as 1991, just before diagnosis, I was still experiencing this feeling of power; the seven dimensions I mentioned. But generally, from the time of breakdown in 1982, the voices became entirely destructive in their content. (Here I must add that I never discuss their intimate content, instead only alluding to general themes. I have always believed that to do so would given them a credence they did not deserve.)

Visual hallucinations are quite terrifying. The nights in my life when I would lie in bed watching the room spark with electricity – a kind of blue fog – upset me greatly. They seemed more frequent when medication was withdrawn.

Disturbance of the sense of smell I have spoken of; again this is very confusing. Like many other hallucinations its effect was to remove me back to times past, a confusing and baffling experience, and invariably negative. It provoked great unhappiness.

Tactile hallucinations, the feeling of touching or being touched by something that is not there, and gustatory hallucinations – things not tasting as they should – are both in themselves disabling. The latter can easily be construed as being somehow poisoned, quite a common delusion.

The point to be made about hallucinations is really the fear that they engender. We all rely on the stability of our surroundings and what goes on in them. If these perceptions become distorted, then the feeling of madness invariably must occur. A case is sometimes made that people who hear voices or have visions are somehow more creative. Certainly it is sometimes possible to utilize the experiences, but history is littered with psychotics who while very artistic in their field suffered enormously. William Blake, Vincent Van Gogh and Richard Dadd are all examples.

Inside or outside? Internalizing and externalizing

A further point must be made on the subject of hallucinations. The psychiatric profession seems obsessed with whether its clients experience voices or see things inside or outside their heads: so-called true and pseudo hallucinations. An internalizer would be described as somebody who felt their voices came from within themselves, their mind. Often this might be a running commentary on their actions and thoughts. Visions, too, could be equally visible internally, behind the eyes. On the other hand somebody described as an externalizer would describe the aural hallucinations as coming from outside, for example a whispering in the ear; or in the visual field – the seeing of things through rather than behind the eyes.

I dispute this rather dogmatic viewpoint, for the simple reason that has, I hope, been shown earlier, that I have experiences of both forms of hallucinations. Nothing is certain in this area; but one point has to be made. My externalized hallucinations have always come at times of increased stress and anxiety. Perhaps there is a link there.

A further point I feel is appropriate. The content and nature of specifical voices is unique to every person with a psychiatric illness. However, the most troubling of aural hallucinations is what are commonly known as command voices – being told to do things, such as harm either to the self or others. Here we enter a more dangerous and sinister world. I suspect that the headline-hitting actions of a schizophrenia sufferer who harms somebody are related to this particular form of distress.

Diminish the positive, accentuate the negative: voices or lethargy?

Many psychotics exhibit florid behaviour when in a voice-hearing phase. This is often perceived as the factor that must be tackled, and the role of medication cannot be either decried or denied. These positive symptoms can in many cases be treated through the use of drugs, with varying degrees of success; however, some people will always be impossible to help in this way.

There are a number of pertinent points to be made on this issue. Again from a personal viewpoint, the distress that positive symptoms engender is quite awful; so the psychiatrist is right to attempt to control them. But there are two issues here to be looked at; one is the medication itself, and particularly its side effects. The other is a common misconception that psychosis itself can be broken down into two types, one where positive symptoms predominate, and the other where negative symptoms are to the fore. Again, I dispute this. Medication might be effective in controlling voices or visions; but how many times does the professional see, either on the ward or in the community, clients who sit blankly all day, overweight and smoking heavily?

And how many turn to drink or drugs to relieve the monotony? Work is denied to many if not most service users; attendance at day hospitals or other therapeutic sessions may be spasmodic and ultimately unsatisfactory.

The fact is that medication is often to blame. Certainly in older, typical medication, negative symptoms are never usually improved and there are often other, physical side effects to be endured. Lethargy, lack of motivation and depression are all common. Even with the new atypicals such as clozapine these functions are still not restored – and here I speak from my own personal experience. Factors such as unemployment are destructive to self-esteem; often the client has lost contact with friends and family, who do not understand his or her condition. This applied to me, particularly with my family, who could not accept my diagnosis. I sank very low indeed. I call this social deskilling, the state whereby the client no longer has the ability or even the desire to partake in social situations. Paranoia can also affect this, making the housebound circumstance of many an inevitability. The empty hours stretch before us. Carers often get frustrated with a client whom they see as doing nothing at all; my partner felt this, the frustration of coming home to find no food on the table in a house that smelt of cigarettes.

Negative symptoms are difficult to shift, undoubtedly. I have built around me a team of consultant, CPN and OTs whose visits and sessions are often the only contact I have outside my main relationship. What friends I had are gone, and I feel still very isolated. Even now, negative feelings often overwhelm me. Depression is inevitable, often coupled with regrets about a lost life.

We are not offered much, turned out into the community only to find it doesn't really care at all. Negativity should be seen for what it is, ultimately very destructive. Mental health professionals should see (and are beginning to see) that diminishing positive symptoms is only half the job. The task now is to complete the job.

Nursing the demons: the biological and environmental components of schizophrenia

This is an area I feel very strongly about. There seems to be an element of confusion as to whether psychosis has as its root cause a chemical imbalance in the brain, or is a product of the upbringing the individual had. This latter viewpoint has in the past led to the blaming or families for a sufferer of schizophrenia's problems; take the client out of the family and they will recover. This is both degrading for all concerned and ultimately destructive; luckily it is a concept that is losing credence.

From my own standpoint, I have developed very clear views from my own evaluation of what has occurred in my life. I believe I have, like many if not all sufferers, a biological predisposition to psychosis. My feelings have suggested for many years that my brain and senses do not function properly (the nights of the blue sparks again). But this still does not mean that I was destined for a schizophrenic breakdown (or at least be so disabled by psychosis). Why it occurred I think is because I grew up in an environment that acted like a hot-house for its development. Socially insecure, in my class as well as with my peers, I learnt to turn my back on the world. As the years passed it became obvious to others that I was becoming stranger. By the time I reached my early twenties, completely withdrawn and not in control of my emotions (I often became angry and broke things) the warning bells should have been sounding.

This combination of predisposition and environment culminated, as I believe it often does, in the facts of my disintegration. I lost sight of who or what I was. (Interestingly, as another issue, the higher incidence of schizophrenic breakdown in certain groups, such as the homeless, those in poverty or prison and various cultural minorities, suggests a strong environmental component.)

Impostors: psychosis as perceptual disorder

My CPN tells me a story of the time she changed her hair colour and then went to visit a client. The client refused to let her in, believing that she was not who she purported to be. It is a simple but actually quite logical tale. I have related the story of when my partner's father came to see me, and I could not believe he was really the man I knew. These two incidents have set me thinking as to why they occurred. Surely it is illogical, a further symptom: after all, the concept of believing in impostors is a documented product of psychotic illness.

So where is the logic? The answer lies in another quite realistic assessment: that schizophrenia involves a distortion of the senses. This I suppose is a biological argument, but I make no apology for it. It occurred to me at a time of great stress, when my perceptions of anything would be out of kilter. Similarly, I had olfactory hallucinations at a period of deep introspection when I was greatly troubled by past life events and circumstances. Visions, too – certainly externalized ones, like the times I saw saints emerging from the bedroom curtains – could be explained in this manner of sensory disruption. Externalized voices have taken place at similar times, often coming with visual distortion. The internalized pattern of experience – inside the head – also seems related to this concept. Voices seemed to become louder when I was put under strain, particularly in public places. Often I could not cope because I could no longer trust my senses – a trust which if lost is at once damning and disabling.

Symptom or coping strategy: the paradigm of withdrawal

You withdraw: therefore you are ill. This perception is a common one. Withdrawal is taken as yet another symptom of mental illness, to be treated along with others. And yet this is a very short-sighted view. I had no conception that my withdrawal was in any way a sign that I was ill. Yes, I admit it was a fact that grew more uncomfortable as I grew older. But I offer another view. People withdraw as a means of coping with their psychosis; it is often the only tool they are left with. I withdrew into my own, virtual world because there I had a level of control that I was losing in reality.

That it became eventually so disturbing was not because it was a symptom, rather that this personal space became progressively invaded by voices and such like. In the years before diagnosis I used to do deals with my hallucinations, allowing them periods of control if they gave me some time where I could withdraw. Some clients report that they miss their voices, a view I can subscribe to. Withdrawal is to me a form of distraction and, as such, should be treated not as symptomatic of illness but a reason to explore the negative cognitions that engender it. Distraction as a technique is often propounded as useful. Do not underestimate this very potent form of distraction: some can only cope by using it.

Rationalizing the irrational: the logic of delusions

For many, the delusions inherent in psychosis are the most difficult factor to understand, both for professionals and for society in general. Because they present as something inherently nonsensical, their treatment is regarded as difficult. But as a client who has suffered from several delusions – initially that I was somehow special, then that I was evil and finally of persecution – I have attempted to analyse the reasons behind them.

In fact, there is logic behind this. Most if not all delusions have roots in real experience, and are often triggered by events. Because I was a bright child intellectually in advance of my peers, it was quite logical to assume that I was special. Equally, coping with the unhappiness of my parents with me and my failure to meet their constant expectations led to a sense that I was just plain bad and a person who could only disappoint and hurt others. There was a devil in me. Finally, someone who was ridiculed by peer groups from the age of 3 until his mid twenties would quite naturally assume he was persecuted; and become paranoid and deluded in any social circumstances.

Analysing the nature of a person's hallucinations is often a way in for the professional. Always there is a logic to this. Perhaps it is the nature of hallucinations that lie behind some delusions: if a man is told constantly by his voices that he is Jesus, he will quite naturally begin to feel that this is true: delusions of grandeur then occur. CBT is a useful tool in the way that it explores the nature of delusions and can often find their trigger. Thus the irrational can become rational; and this is far easier to deal with.

Look for the logic of delusions; do not see them as merely deranged symptoms. This means a client can be treated far more as a human being and less as an illness.

A client's guide to schizophrenia: the five stages of psychotic experience

Moving on from the deluded world, my life-events have encouraged me to try to gain a measure of how my symptoms relate to one another, above all in the order they present. They fall into five clear stages (see Figure 1.1). The first, and in many ways the easiest but still annoying to deal with, is thought echo. This, like hearing your own thoughts, often as a running commentary, is always for me the precursor to later stages of schizophrenic symptoms. These continue into a second phase, which is sometimes referred to as a 'stream of consciousness'. Personally I find this quite disabling, because it involves a

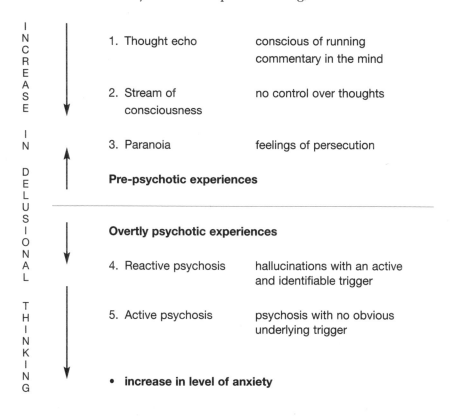

Figure 1.1 Five stages of psychotic experience

filling up of the mind with recollected dreams, all sinister and distorted, and these run at great speed through my conscious being. My partner asked what this term meant; unable to understand my somewhat garbled explanation, she came up with the best description of it that I have ever heard. She asked if it was like trying to get to sleep but being unable to, with your mind racing away, thoughts all running into one another. Again this is disabling, particularly when it occurs at times of stress or in public situations.

The third area is a crucial point. In Figure 1.1 I have shown these first phases as pre-psychotic symptoms, because I believe that we can all experience them, mentally ill or not. Take the case of paranoia. I question whether many people have not experienced this at some period in their life: waiting for exam results (I have failed. What can I do? People will laugh at me) or the letter after that job interview. We all at some time feel this panic. It is a way in for professionals: surely it is easier to engage with a client if they themselves have understood these early symptoms.

The fourth and fifth phases represent a breakdown of what might best be described as overtly psychiatric symptoms. First there comes what I call reactive psychosis. This is a level of symptoms which are all previously documented: but the crucial fact is that they occur with an identifiable trigger, such as busy places or a room where something disturbing occurred previously. These triggers, when explored, can be mitigated, I feel, and the effect of the hallucinations can perhaps be lessened. This leads on to the worst phase, what I term active psychosis. This is an onset of symptoms without an underlying trigger, perhaps in a place of security such as home or even hospital. From my previous comments from a personal point of view I hope to have shown that these present as an externalized force.

Throughout these levels there is an increase both in delusional thinking and in levels of anxiety.

The head versus the heart: medication and compliance

Recently, as I have said, I became involved in teaching mental health professionals about psychosis. There is a heavy emphasis on role-play in this course; I usually portray a client who is still disturbed. However, on one occasion I was asked to respond to the questions in my real persona. The assessment we were doing was the Drug Attitude Index (the DAI 30). This little survey tests a client's responses and attitudes to medication. In my head I have always known that I needed drugs to be well (at least in the past seven years, but not previously as I have said). Logically, therefore, I should have responded positively in my answers to questions such as 'do you feel you need to take medication?' and 'does medication make you feel better?' But my truest answers were negative; though intellectually I knew that I needed medication, my instincts were that I did not want to take it.

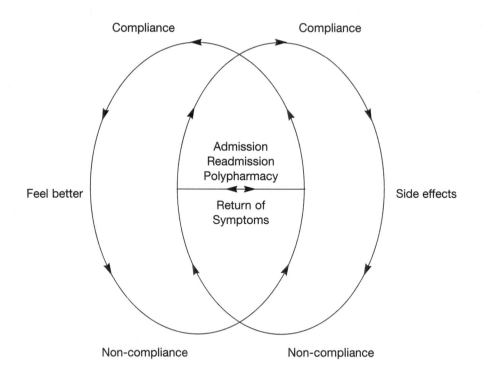

Figure 1.2 Issues of compliance

This throws up an interesting dilemma. I still have great reservations about medication. In fact I feel confused. It leads on to the issues of compliance and non-compliance, which I can best represent in a diagram (Figure 1.2) which I call the circles of non-compliance. Simply, there are two major reasons why clients stop taking their drugs. The first is that they feel better. This is a point of education; it must be imparted to people that medication works only if it is continued: it is not like taking paracetamol for a headache. The second is the thorny issue of side effects. If these are too severe and distressing, then it is quite logical to stop taking what is causing them. Both circles meet and lead to identical processes – a return of symptoms, admission or readmission or polypharmacy. It is a negative spiral that must, I feel, be addressed.

Medication is one of the most complicated areas in the treatment of mental illness. My own thoughts are, that with modern, atypical drugs with far fewer side effects, compliance can increase. If I were a doctor, I could never give a person pills that I knew would cause terrible distress, however effective they were in treating overt symptoms. They should be consigned to history.

CBT and the art of desymptomizing

This title uses a word that, although ugly, best describes my own experience of therapy other than medication. It is no exaggeration to say it altered my entire outlook on life. First, though, my symptoms had to be reduced, for CBT as a process cannot work if the client is in too much distress. Effective drugs opened up new possibilities, but they could not have worked on their own. My interpretation of CBT is that it challenges patterns of thinking; if you are ill, therefore you think ill. To feel well again, you must think well. There are practical assessments of mental state to be gone through, such as the Manchester Scale, the DAI 30 mentioned previously and the rather long-winded Liverpool University Neuroleptic Side-effect Ratings Scale, abbreviated (thankfully!) as LUNSERS. These assessments are useful in gauging where a client is in their treatment; in addition, some result in scores which can be monitored if the process is repeated sometime later – a tangible tool to measure improvement or worsening of a situation.

For me personally, my architectural training and perceptions – I think in terms of buildings, their aspects, lightness and the security they offer – were used. I drew houses and bridges, and formalized my thinking. I realized I thought in circles, unable to break out of negative thinking. By interrupting these circles, it was possible to control any symptoms that broke though medication. There are still times when I sense that I am going to be ill: but now instead of descending into psychosis, I know I do not have to. I leave the circle of schizophrenic behaviour. Desymptomizing is the best way I can describe it. It breaks the self-fulfilling prophecy that is psychosis: it first isolates the sufferer, then feeds on that isolation.

The carer in the community

As I draw to a close, I must make a point about the role and frequent mistreatment of those who look after a person with mental illness. I have a partner who has stayed with me throughout this time; quite simply I could not have survived without her. She has shown great fortitude and love, despite my best efforts when very ill to push her away. But she has been most sorely treated by the services. Initially she sought to inform herself of my condition, and guide me through the maze of diagnosis and treatment. Gradually however, with time she has been marginalized and her views disregarded, particularly in the incident of ECT. Many carers I feel sure can relate to this frustration. They are unsung heroes who save the health service a vast amount of money. They should be treated with respect.

Endgame: recovery and beyond

Finally, I end with an assessment of this work. I wrote at the start of my desire to convey something of the life of a man who has for most of his life been, in the bluntest of terms, mentally ill. But I have survived; and still, after many setbacks, believe fundamentally that treatment is best offered by the service of doctors and other professionals. But it is a service, and we have the right as clients to expect it to be as good as possible.

Many factors in my story obviously contribute to the strength and depth of my problems: difficult upbringing, inability to relate to others and late presentation.

But now I am recovering; not an easy process, but one that I hope I have shown can be held out for others. We are not mad; but we need help. If given, the chances for many will improve. That is the hope I cling to.

I return eventually to my title: the science of enduring madness. I have been there and am now coming back. I have endured the trials and pitfalls of a disturbing life that could have been totally destroyed by schizophrenia. But my life is now enduring: it goes on.

Slowly, surely, I live again. In the words of T.S. Eliot again, in the conclusion to *East Coker*:

In my end is my beginning.

CHAPTER TWO

A carer's view of schizophrenia

RONALD W. RYALL

Schizophrenia is usually a devastating experience not only for the person with the illness (the sufferer[1]) but for the whole family. In this chapter I review the definition of carers of people with schizophrenia and examine the role that carers can and often should play, their concerns about the illness and its effect on the person they care for, that person's future life and, last but not least, the impact of schizophrenia on carers themselves and their relationships. Within the concept of a holistic approach to the care of people with schizophrenia, the perceptions, contributions and burdens of carers cannot be ignored.

Who cares?

The importance of understanding the role of carers as the best informants, as those frequently providing the majority of the community and psychological support and as those maintaining continuity of support over long periods (often a lifetime) for those with schizophrenia cannot be overemphasized. Professionals often perceive carers of people with schizophrenia only as those who are closely related or with whom the person is living. This is an oversimplification that can lead to unjustified assumptions, sometimes leading to serious or even disastrous consequences, especially when information is sought in relation to risk assessment.

Rhona Sergeant (1993) concluded

> ...it would seem that little has changed in nearly twenty years... Communication between health professionals and relatives is poor, relatives would prefer to be treated as part of the multidisciplinary team, and there is a need for general education about schizophrenia.

---

[1] Although the use of the word 'sufferer', as applied to a person with schizophrenia, in some ways misrepresents the illness, it is a convenient and much-used term and, in the absence of a suitably brief alternative, will be used throughout this chapter.

Several years on from that, I conclude that although there has been considerable progress in ideology and strategy there has been considerably less progress in implementation. This volume may help to bridge some of that gap.

This chapter therefore begins with consideration of the broader concept of 'who cares?'

Statutory carers

Traditionally, professionals in the statutory agencies, including health and social services, tend to view themselves as the major providers of treatment and information in relation to serious mental illness such as schizophrenia. Historically, little was done in clinical practice to help carers face the considerable burdens which they bear as carers of people with functional illness (Kuipers and Bebbington 1985). These authors drew attention to the fact that not only did relatives deserve and need help but they could also be used as an effective resource in the management of patients with severe functional illness, especially schizophrenia.

Increasingly, especially in the 1990s, development of the government's Care Programme Approach (Department of Health 1990, 1994, 1999a) has changed the emphasis in strategy, but carers' perceptions of actual practice have sometimes changed little over that period, and in many cases the outcome falls far short of the ideal (see also report from the Social Services Inspectorate 1998). The growing development of community mental health teams providing regular input to individuals over long periods has helped to change implementation a little, but these teams are vastly under-resourced. New trends in organization, commissioning and implementation of mental health programmes, spurred on by the *National Service Framework for Mental Health* (Department of Health 1999b) and programmes such as *Effective Care Co-ordination in Mental Health Services: Modernising the Care Programme Approach* (Department of Health 1999a), the *New NHS Plan* (Department of Health 2000a) and major reviews of structural organization currently in progress should help to change the perception and implementation of high quality care. The past model of provision solely by all-powerful, all-knowing professionals is now increasingly rare, and is slowly but surely changing to that of an equal partnership between professional carers and other carers in giving support and treatment in its widest sense, and friendship and advice to those with schizophrenia and other psychotic disorders. Such changes were recommended long ago in the comprehensive advisory document *Building Bridges* (Department of Health 1995), which gives much pertinent and detailed advice about working together between professional agencies, formal and informal carers and the voluntary sector working for the care and protection of mentally ill people.

National independent sector organizations such as the National Schizophrenia Fellowship (NSF), Manic Depression Fellowship, MIND and SANE, have had a major impact on strategy and awareness of the wider implications of user and carer involvement. In addition, some, such as the NSF and MIND, now directly provide a variety of services ranging from advocacy through residential care to employment, and other day care provision. The NSF, originally set up to provide support groups for carers, continues to be the major support group for carers of people with severe mental illness.

The 'new' approach should yield a holistic view of the needs of people with schizophrenia that should lessen the absolute dependence on medication and the doctor or the GP, although these three will inevitably remain the first lines of defence for the foreseeable future.

Informal carers

As opposed to the 'formal' carers in the statutory agencies, there is that vast array of other carers who are often little heeded. This includes not just relatives, but those in other relationships, such as employers and friends. Often overlooked, but providing an essential element of continuing care for many people with schizophrenia who are unable to sustain independent living in the community, are those care workers in supported housing, especially those in registered residential care homes, who may constitute the major care, support and friendship for some of their clients.

Relationships of carers who have joined the mailing list and have sought help from the NSF support group in Cambridge over a period of about 15 years are analysed in Table 2.1. The data on 392 carers were extracted from a database maintained by the author.

Table 2.1 Relationship between 392 carers and the sufferer

Relation of sufferer to carer	Percentage of total
Son	42.0
Daughter	18.0
Brother	11.0
Husband	7.9
Sister	5.9
Friend	5.0
Mother	3.8
Wife	3.6
Father	1.8
Partner	0.5
Others	0.5

Since the peak age of first incidence of schizophrenia, especially in men, is 18–25 years, it is not surprising that the majority of carers at that time are parents. This also leads to the conclusion that most carers, except for siblings and children, will range in age upwards from about 45 years. However, to assume that always to be the case is to miss the great variety of human interactions which are important for the support and care of the person with schizophrenia.

It is notable that in almost all gender pairs, for example, son–daughter, husband–wife, but with the exception of the mother–father relationship, male sufferers outnumber female sufferers by a factor of two. It is known that the numbers of men and women with schizophrenia are about equal. One factor that could explain the discrepancy may be that the severity or nature of the illness in men, especially young men, may lead more of their carers to come forward. In addition, it has been a prominent feature of the author's experience in running a support group that a greater preponderance of women come forward as the principal carer, compared with men who often stand more apart from this direct role. The mother–father discrepancy is more difficult to explain. One possibility is that when a parent has schizophrenia, the offspring are more concerned about the mother, who has been the principal carer, than the father. It is otherwise unclear why this should be so.

There are many other types of caring roles ranging from heterosexual and homosexual partnerships to friends and family, including children, parents, siblings, more distant relations, teachers and counsellors. The problems and anxieties generated in each of these groups have many factors in common but there are also particular concerns associated with the particular relationships that are often ignored or are not given the opportunity to be revealed. These individual needs and concerns of carers will be examined in this chapter.

The Nearest Relative

The Nearest Relative is a legal description arising from the Mental Health Act 1983. It is not synonymous with next of kin. The term is likely to be removed from new legislation arising from the White Paper on the reform of the Mental Health Act published in December 2000[2], and will be replaced by new carers' rights which should remove some of the anomalies of the current system and give further protection to patients.

---

[2] In September 2002 the Government published a 'Draft Mental Health Bill and Consultation Document'. However, various aspects of this draft produced such strong opposition from the Royal College of Psychiatrists and other organizations that the new bill did not appear in the Queen's speech at the end of 2002. Informal assurance has been given that the final Bill will include important changes in content to reflect the strong views put forward during the consultation stage about various aspects of the proposals. However, there is no definite news as yet (January 2003).

Case study – Mrs A

Ms A is a single parent. Her son, aged 28, lives with her. He has not worked for five years. He has no diagnosis but she thinks that it is schizophrenia and this is certainly highly likely. The symptoms have not been followed up by the GP, who has been rather less than helpful.

The son is now deluded. She will not let him know she has contacted the NSF because she is fearful of the reaction.

Issues:

- How should she be advised about seeking the help that is so clearly needed?
- Should she be encouraged to continue to contact the NSF secretly?

We did not feel in the circumstances that we should advise her simply to go away and only do more when matters had reached breaking point. In the event the NSF helped her to obtain the necessary intervention, which proceeded smoothly.

Carers' perceptions of the problems of schizophrenia

It is significant that carers and users attribute priorities to the problems they encounter that are different from those of the professionals who are responsible for assessment of their needs. A number of studies over many years have all yielded comparable results. Creer and Wing (1975) listed the frequency of problems reported by carers, as shown in Table 2.2.

Table 2.2 Carers' perceptions of schizophrenia (Creer and Wing 1975)

Problem	Frequency (%)	Problem	Frequency (%)
Social withdrawal	74	Odd movements	25
Underactivity	56	Threats of violence	25
Lack of conversation	54	Poor mealtime behaviour	13
Few leisure interests	50	Socially embarrassing	8
Slowness	48	Sexually unusual	8
Overacting	41	Suicide attempts	4
Odd ideas/behaviour	34	Incontinence	4
Depression	34		

In a survey of 886 members of the NSF, Tyler (1979, unpublished) produced similar results (Table 2.3).

Table 2.3 Carers' perceptions of schizophrenia (Tyler 1979, unpublished)

Problem	Frequency (%)
Lack of motivation/indecision	69
Depression/anxiety	49
Withdrawal/lying in bed	45
Neglect of hygiene/appearance	36
Violent outbursts from frustration	30
Food problems	14

It is significant that the problems that most worry carers are not the positive symptoms, which are those most amenable to medication, but the negative symptoms, which are relatively resistant. In recent times, major concerns reported by carers still concentrate on lack of motivation and drive, accounting for many of the symptoms listed above, and social dysfunction. Carers request support organizations for increasingly more detailed comparative information and advice about medication. However, there has been much more emphasis on obesity – an effect of all antipsychotic drugs – and sexual dysfunction. Interestingly, the major problems reported by the users are generally not so different from those reported by carers, with even more emphasis on the negative effects of medication.

The differences in perceptions between professional carers, users and informal carers are also highlighted in a report entitled *Relative Values* (Shepherd, Murray and Muijen 1994), a study carried out by the Sainsbury Centre for Mental Health.

The lessons from these observations should be clear: in treating schizophrenia it is necessary to place far more emphasis on the socially disabling effects of the illness and of medication, including weight gain, and not to rely entirely on the more favourable outcome in relation to positive symptoms such as 'voices'. It is all too easy and much less resource intensive just to prescribe medication. Since it is easier to achieve a reduction of positive symptoms than of negative symptoms, despite the perceived greater importance of the latter, it is understandable that the professional carers will derive more immediate satisfaction from focusing on the more readily treatable positive symptoms. There is a strong need for training of staff in this area to change the cultural thrust of the care programme.

Stages of caring

The consequence of making false general assumptions – that carers all need the same support, advice and information at the same time – is unhelpful and can be counterproductive.

The input that carers need and the demands that can be put upon them will vary according to the stage in the development or recovery from the illness, the severity and nature of symptoms, the effectiveness or otherwise of treatment and the particular aptitudes, interests, concerns, anxieties and abilities of the carers. Carers' active involvement as contributors to the care programme for the person they love and care for is essential if their contribution is to be helpful. The need for them to be consulted as equal partners wherever possible should be recognized and implemented. Mere token adherence to good practice guidelines is insufficient.

It is convenient to group needs according to the stages in the illness. However, the comments about individual differences in need mentioned above should be remembered.

Pre-diagnostic

The diagnosis of schizophrenia is generally made in the late teens or early twenties. However, parents often detect major problems before a diagnosis is made, even before any medical advice is sought. The behavioural problems may be attributed to the problems of adolescence. This is not necessarily to be discouraged, because the dangers of inaccurate early diagnosis may outweigh the benefits. Nevertheless, there are some who favour an early diagnosis and treatment on the grounds that such early intervention may prevent the degree or speed of development of the illness. Until the predictability of treatment outcomes and accuracy of diagnoses can be assured, there is a good argument for the view that the greater advantage is to be obtained by allowing as normal development as possible, with the maximum possible degree of independence. This will allow a better prognosis for subsequent rehabilitation and recovery following relapse.

Most parents now have some elementary knowledge about the symptoms of schizophrenia and often, in my experience, make their own diagnosis long before they are given one by the GP or psychiatrist. It is understandable why doctors are reluctant to make early diagnoses because of the stigma that persists around the label of schizophrenia. Nevertheless, for many sufferers and their carers the delivering of a clear and fully explained diagnosis can greatly ease the anxieties and burdens. To know what the problem is and to have it identified to them implies that medical knowledge will then have the means to alleviate the symptoms. This is better for the development of confidence in professional care than the uncertainty of the professionals being unable to identify the problem and therefore unable to propose a treatment.

These contradictory approaches must be resolved, and at some point a diagnosis must be attempted and the outcome conveyed to anxious sufferers and carers. Sometimes, the psychiatrist has already made a diagnosis but does not wish to worry a carer unduly or prematurely. This is misguided.

Even before a formal diagnosis is made, the carer will derive great benefit from talking to other, experienced carers of those with established diagnoses, provided those other carers can appreciate the uncertainties that exist at that time. The experienced carers will have positive outcomes to relate, as well as a more pragmatic approach to the immediate problems. I have always been surprised that the prognoses given by psychiatrists to carers in the early stages of pre-diagnosis and diagnosis are so pessimistic.

Case study – Mrs B

Mrs B is a single parent with a 4-year-old child. She has a brother-in-law, aged 31, who lives with his parents. He has cut off all friends and sits at home all day doing nothing. He tries to get jobs, but they last for only 2–3 days. He believes everyone is against him and sees things that are not there – it is difficult to be specific. He is periodically verbally abusive, mostly to his parents. The symptoms described, which have persisted for about three years, are almost certainly schizophrenic. The parents have no doctor or diagnosis or help or medication or insight.

Issues

Mrs B is clearly very concerned about the effect of the illness on her brother-in-law and on his parents. She is also anxious about getting herself involved, for obvious reasons.

She wants advice on how to proceed. A number of interesting issues arise here. For example, there is a clear necessity to ease the concern of Mrs B. There is also a need to alert the parents, if possible, to possible actions they could take, or where they could go for support and advice if they feel that they need it. There is also a clear possibility of premature early intervention which may exacerbate the problems.

Early post-diagnostic

The immediate impact of a diagnosis of schizophrenia, particularly if delivered 'out of the blue', sometimes without further explanation, and usually without the offer of support or steering towards support agencies, can be devastating for carers. Even if they have already guessed the diagnosis, the actual delivery can have an equally great effect. All too often the immediate questions are unanswered. These questions will most likely relate to:

- What will happen next?
- What hope is there for the future?
- What do I do?

Other questions will come later.

The carer will most likely already have become familiar with the gradual increase in tension in the family, the impact of mental illness on other family members, the decreasing functioning of the person just diagnosed. However, they will rarely have come to terms with the sudden changing of expectations and aspirations which usually accompany the diagnosis, usually following extreme and acute breakdown.

This sudden apparent 'loss of the person they knew', coupled with a need to adapt to a new set of expectations, has been likened to bereavement after the death of a close relative or friend. The period of bereavement may follow a different time course in different people, but there is always a need for counselling and support. Usually, the carers feel isolated and alone, grappling with a problem to which no one seems to have adequate answers or explanations.

Carers need at this time to have their hopes and aspirations set, if anything, on the high side. With the passage of time it may be necessary to adapt to more realistic and lower expectations of recovery or rehabilitation. Only too frequently, under the guise of setting realistic expectations, excessively pessimistic outcomes are conveyed to carers who may become exceedingly depressed as a consequence. The effect of this is to reduce their ability to cope with the changed circumstances and to help the sufferer.

Some of the particular feelings experienced by carers are addressed in the next section, 'The burden of caring'.

During hospital admission

A hospital admission is often associated with the first severe breakdown. For those who have been on an acute admission ward many times, it is difficult to remember how traumatic this can be for the carer, let alone the sufferer. For most it will be the first experience of seeing a number of mentally unwell people at the same time in the same, partially restricted and disturbed environment, all in a state of relapse, and many of them heavily drugged. Fortunately, hospital ward environments are currently undergoing vast improvements and ward culture towards carers is slowly changing for the better.

It is therefore of the utmost importance that the communication skills of staff are such that they can alleviate anxieties by explaining the nature and philosophy of the care that they will be providing, and the likely duration of the stay. It is also necessary to give some clear guidelines to carers about visiting and their roles and involvement while the sufferer is in hospital. At this point some guidance about support organizations and basic information needs must be addressed. Carers must be kept informed of progress, or lack of it. The last thing they want to hear is 'Johnny is doing as well as can be expected' only to discover when they visit that he is in fact exceedingly unwell.

When a person is detained under the Mental Health Act, there are statutory and good practice requirements for carers to be informed of their rights. New legislation is likely to require that their involvement in care plans is outlined soon after admission. At the moment, many professionals comply with good practice simply by giving a brief pamphlet to the carer, when what is required is a detailed explanation to go with it.

At and after discharge

All patients discharged from hospital should now be provided with a detailed care plan as part of the fulfilment of Care Programme Approach protocols. Copies of this care plan should be given to all carers providing a substantial amount of care. Carers should be involved as partners in the development of the care plan, which should give basic information about support and support agencies and organizations, housing, treatment and medication, follow-up support for the sufferer, the name of the care co-ordinator, dates of first follow-up appointments, and contingency plans and contact phone numbers. Many sufferers from schizophrenia will also need information and help in gaining access to benefits and, if required, sheltered housing. Carers should be given clear indications of actions they should take if they feel that help is needed.

If the patient has been detained under the Mental Health Act, then the carer, as well as the sufferer, should be informed about the significance of Section 117 aftercare under the Act, particularly recent legal judgements concerning responsibility for financing in their entirety the residential needs of such ex-patients (Department of Health 2000b).

Long term

Most carers come to terms with and adapt to mental illness of long duration. The early expectations of rapid recovery, cure by effective treatments, return to the life that existed before the illness, expectation of successes in the future in academic or other fields of endeavour will have either been fulfilled if the patient recovered, or only partially or even not at all after many years of ongoing illness with or without repeated hospital admissions.

However, new questions will now arise. The concerns will be more about quality of life issues, or employment at a level that remains stimulating for the sufferer and yet does not make demands beyond his or her capabilities. There will be concerns about the loss of independence that may come from long-term severe mental illness and concerns about how care will be provided for the indefinite future.

Carers will become increasingly concerned about their long-term role as they get older, and about future financial provisions.

The ageing carer

Many carers with their own financial resources will become concerned as they enter their seventies, or even before, about the types of provision that they should make for their families, including the special needs of the person with schizophrenia. It is obvious that the urgency of those needs and the difficulties that may be expected will depend very much upon the mental state, self-confidence, reliability, financial wisdom and independence of the sufferer. This matter is considered in a separate section on wills and trusts.

In addition to financial matters, carers will be increasingly concerned with the question of who will provide the emotional and social support that they have been giving all their lives. This is not easily answered and is inadequately addressed by the organizations responsible for providing care. It is essential that alternative arrangements are put in place early on to lessen the dependence on the ageing carer for financial, psychological and emotional support. These alternatives should range from befriending, through individual professional support from community mental health teams to formal engagement with clubs and out-of-hospital activities of many kinds, including sheltered work at many different levels.

At times, excessive demands are placed upon aging parents, as illustrated in the example below.

Case study – Mr and Mrs C

Mr and Mrs C are the ageing parents of a son who has schizophrenia and a history of lack of insight and non-compliance with medication. He normally lives alone. He was arrested for possession of a large quantity of cannabis, which was not denied. He was taken to court and charged and then released on bail with parental surety, conditional on his living with parents and a 9 p.m. curfew, until sentenced. The parents wanted advice on whether to accept this immense burden and what action they should take to ensure that his mental state was properly taken into consideration.

In the end, because of a sense of responsibility, they accepted the conditions in order to prevent their son going to prison while awaiting sentence. However, it was more than 18 months before sentence was passed.

Issues

- Should ageing parents have been subjected to this type of responsibility by the court, which they clearly did not want?
- Should the time on bail have been made considerably shorter so as to lessen this burden?
- Should the parents have been strongly advised against accepting such bail conditions?

The burden of caring

Caring can be a fulfilling and positive experience both for the carer and the sufferer. It can give value to one's life and to the life of the sufferer. It can also be a negative experience and a burden if it is carried out to an excessive or sometimes obsessive degree. It is a burden if carers feel unable to cope or have unrealistic expectations for the outcome of their efforts.

Burdens of caring can be alleviated by understanding, warmth, empathy, information and the acquisition of special skills and patience and the acceptance of one's limit to care alone. The last of these can be realized only if the additional support required is easily available at a time when it is needed. For this to occur, there needs to be good communication between all carers, both professional and informal.

Kinship and caring

It is a sad fact that most people with schizophrenia do not marry or form other close partnerships. It follows that most informal carers who contribute a substantial amount of care are parents, usually middle aged or elderly.

Where people with schizophrenia do marry or enter long-term relationships, it is the partner who bears the brunt of the caring role. Often in such circumstances the relationship began before the onset of the mental illness and the subsequent decline in mental state is extremely traumatic for the partner. Nevertheless, many stay with the partner and accept the new form of the relationship, especially where there are children. It is particularly difficult for those partners to fulfil themselves. Their devotion, tenacity and often self-sacrifice is to be admired, but rarely do they get adequate recognition or support. Many relationships do not withstand the ravages of severe and enduring schizophrenia.

Guilt, blame and shame

Most carers at first feel a sense of guilt and blame themselves in some way for the illness. Particularly if they are parents, there may be a sense of failure and shame that they appear to have been so inadequate in parenting skills. How many times have I heard it said, 'If only I had done something differently, perhaps this would not have happened!'? This feeling of guilt is often fuelled by the concurrence of some traumatic life event immediately preceding the first, and sometimes subsequent, breakdowns, such as leaving home, death of a family member or marital disharmony, when the carer may feel a sense that they have somehow failed to provide the support required.

The inappropriate feeling of guilt may lead carers to isolate themselves from friends and relations, which is not helpful and can lead to disintegration of the carer as well as the sufferer. The feeling is natural, especially when the breakdown occurs in the late teenage years. It can be countered by good-quality information and advice or even possibly counselling. It is often alleviated by contact with carers from other families and the knowledge that many feel the same way at first. The voice of authority in the person of the psychiatrist or GP is most likely to be the most quickly effective. Equally, the negative messages given by unthinking or poorly informed professionals are the most difficult to counter.

Bereavement

The feeling akin to bereavement experienced by many carers after the first onset of schizophrenia is understandable. The person they have known and loved for so many years, and their relationship with them, seem to them to have vanished. Without hope for the future, the feeling of bereavement will most likely endure. It will be curtailed by the onset of hope and the knowledge and experience to be gained from contact with other carers, together with the personal experience they will gain from the fact of remission in most cases. In the meantime, professional counselling may well be required and should certainly be considered.

Confusion

The rapid breakdown that so often occurs at the first episode of schizophrenia gives no time for carers to adapt to changing circumstances or to acquire new skills and knowledge. The lack of readily available source material catering for their special needs and made available to them at short notice, and a lack of professional advice and information or reluctance to give it, often leads to a state of confusion. This is made worse when the professionals seem unable to make decisions or seem frequently to be changing what they are trying to do. The worst-case scenario is when the professionals involved give conflicting advice or information to the carers. As always, communication is the key to success.

Inadequacy

Many carers have been capable and successful in their own lives. The inability to influence to any significant degree the course of events in the sufferer can lead to a profound sense of failure and inadequacy. The greater the social isolation in the family, the greater will be the sense of inadequacy. Without outside intervention, the vicious circle of events will become self-perpetuating and reinforcing.

Loss of expectations

Parents and partners will, by the very nature of their relationships with their offspring or partners, have developed certain expectations and aspirations for the future of the relationship. Schizophrenia often strikes just as a young person is beginning to realize those potentials, or when a relationship has reached a certain level of satisfaction. The devastating effect of the illness, even in the short term, often leads to the sense of disappointment and frustration in the carer, who feels they can do little to restore the status quo.

There is an oft-quoted maxim that a person who has experienced schizophrenia will never again be the 'same' person. Although this is often self-evident, it is not always appreciated that the person who has or has had schizophrenia is often a person who is more sensitive to the needs of others, quiet and uncomplaining for most of the time and accepting of their circumstances which can hardly be considered to have changed for the better. It may take carers a long time to appreciate this positive side of schizophrenia but most will, in the fullness of time, come to lower their sights and set expectations and aspirations at a realistic level.

Disempowerment

Close carers will have been, for long time, in a position to influence and help the person they care for. When that person becomes ill, they continue to care, with or without the necessary skills. When all care is then taken over by professionals, and carers are excluded from involvement with the process or decision-making (which may itself make assumptions about their own involvement), the feeling of disempowerment can itself have a detrimental effect on the health of the carer.

Alienation

Alienation can occur at two levels: alienation from the sufferer and alienation from the professional carers.

Some carers will experience a sense of alienation from a person with schizophrenia, especially when that person has persistent delusional paranoid ideas about the carer. These may vary from extreme cases where the carer experiences extreme hostility or is perceived, for example, to be poisoning the sufferer or at least causing them harm or interfering in their affairs unnecessarily. Only the experience of knowing that this state does not usually persist will diminish the sense of alienation.

Carers often feel alienated by doctors, nurses and social workers who misguidedly view the sufferer as their sole focus of attention, ignoring the consequences for the family. This occurs less frequently now than it did just a few years ago, but there is still a problem in some areas. To a great degree the improvement can be attributed to the growing influence of carer organizations on the culture of professional care, and on government policy which has become markedly more carer-positive over the years.

Of course, it must be accepted that there are some rare occasions when the involvement of the family or carer should be limited in the interests of the patient. However, lack of involvement can be more usually attributed to poor practice.

Stigma

Stigma is the negative imputation that is attached to a person's reputation. The consequences of stigmatization are prolific, having social, psychological and practical consequences. Stigmatization is often ill informed and judgements misguided. Unfortunately, mental illness, particularly schizophrenia, has been poorly served in this respect by the media, which often portrays the person with schizophrenia as a menace to society, if not dangerous to the person, while failing to reveal the norm as a shy retiring person, often socially and economically deprived as a consequence of illness. The stigma of mental illness also rubs off on the carers. They may try to hide the illness from close friends or even close relatives. Not only does this produce an intolerable strain on relationships, but it is exceedingly stressful for the carer. Although the reality of the stigma does have a major impact on the ability of the sufferer to integrate with society and to find employment, the fact of mental illness should not impair the social life of the carer. Many carers come to realize this only by contact with other carers who have managed to combine their caring role with an otherwise fairly normal lifestyle. However, it must also be recognized that if the carer receives inadequate support then there will be a negative effect on the life of that carer.

Impact on employment

A major concern of carers is for the future employment of the sufferer. There is certainly too little provision for gainful employment at an appropriate level.

Less evident is that in some cases there is also a negative impact of the illness on the employment of a carer. This can easily arise when the employee's performance suffers as a consequence of worries and anxieties about the care of the person with schizophrenia. If the carer is a major contributor to day-to-day care, which takes a large part of their time, there will obviously be an adverse effect on their ability to undertake paid employment.

﹏ng with suicide

﹏, perhaps most, close carers of those with schizophrenia have to face ﹏ear or even the reality of suicide attempts or of death though suicide. ﹏co-ordinator of a local support group, I have encountered this situ-﹏ repeatedly over the years among my clients. It is salutary to ﹏mber that one person in every 10 with schizophrenia may actually kill ﹏selves (Hogman and Meier 1995).

﹏e instinctive first reaction of carers to threats of suicide is panic and ﹏l-enveloping protectiveness. Often, they are the first to learn of the sui-﹏ thoughts but in the absence of good communication with the ﹏essional advisers who are knowledgeable about the sufferer, they have ﹏esource to turn to, unless they are fortunate enough to be in contact ﹏ a support group that has experience of such matters. If the suicide ﹏increases while the person is a patient in hospital, relatives are often ﹏informed about it until there has been a serious incident. To be unpre-﹏ed is a recipe for excessive reactions – even disaster if communication ﹏ischarge or when granting leave of absence is poor or absent, as is so ﹏n the case.

﹏he importance of gathering information from informants, including ﹏tives and carers, has been emphasized repeatedly in inquiry reports ﹏o homicide and suicide.

﹏tandard 7 of the *National Service Framework* (Department of Health ﹏9b) is about decreasing the incidence of suicide. One way to contribute ﹏lowering risk is to increase communication with the carers, both in the ﹏ly stages of admission, in order to obtain historical facts and experi-﹏ces from the carers, and during admission and before discharge. Carers ﹏ould always contribute to risk assessment.

Case study – Mr and Mrs E

Mr and Mrs E had a schizophrenic son who had been very ill but gained insight after effective treatment. He became very depressed. Tragically, he committed suicide while he was in a relatively insightful state in which he had carefully and realistically appraised the consequences of his ill-ness on his life and potential.

Issue

Is enough support and counselling given to people who regain insight after effective treatment, following prolonged periods of severe mental illness, causing high levels of non-functioning?

Impact of caring on carers' relationships

It has been the author's experience that the male pa[r]
often leave the major burden of care to the women.
for a while into the neutral atmosphere of the workp
not the case for women, especially if they are mother[s]

The different caring roles adopted by the partner[s]
ences of view about care, to marital tensions an[d]
breakdown. This is more likely to occur when the care[r]
fessional support and involvement that is needed.

Coping with drug addiction (dual diagnosis)

Perhaps one of the most difficult matters for parents to
is drug addiction in someone with schizophrenia. Here
between respect for the law and the mitigating factor o[f]
ness. Many carers in this situation are extremely caring a[nd]
more professional carers are not. I have encountered ex[amples of individ]
uals with severe mental illness being evicted by their land[lords because]
of drug taking and of patients being discharged from c[are/deten]
tion, purely to enable them to be arrested and charged
drug charges.

More enlightened policies are required for dealing wit[h this increasing]
ly prevalent problem.

Case study – Mr and Mrs D

Mr and Mrs D's son, who normally lives at home with th[em, was admit]
ted to hospital on Section 3. He has a dual diagn[osis (drug abuse and]
schizophrenia).

He was discharged from Section 3 at short notice with[out notifying]
the parents and arrested by the police in hospital on the s[ame day. The]
police were notified by the hospital. When Mr and Mrs D[   ]
they were told that it was not hospital practice to notify re[latives of dis]
charge.

Issues

- Section 133 of the Mental Health Act requires Nearest R[elative to be]
  notified in advance of discharge from detention under th[e Act.]
- Hospital policy was changed.
- Clear policies are required to be followed when drugs ar[e found]
  in hospital.

Confidentiality

Whenever the suggestion of increased communication with carers is raised, the matter of 'confidentiality' arises. However, carers often contrast the behaviour and communication of nurses and doctors in relation to mental illness with the behaviour of similar professionals in other areas of medicine. For example, it is an almost universal experience that when a person is in intensive care or undergoing almost any form of major surgery, then confidentiality seems not be an issue. Indeed, in most cases when the issue is approached with sufferers from mental illness in a positive fashion, explaining the benefits of good communication, then there is rarely a problem with 'confidentiality'.

Case study – Mrs F

Mrs F had a son who lived independently far away in his own flat. From telephone contacts, she was aware that he was suicidal. He was found overdosed by his landlord and taken to Accident and Emergency. The landlord informed the mother by telephone. She called the A&E department to inform them of her fears and to ask them to keep him in hospital (i.e. detain him under the Mental Health Act): she was the Nearest Relative, although this was not accepted by the hospital. A&E refused to talk to her on grounds of confidentiality. It appears that they also mistakenly believed, despite her protestations, that she was the patient's sister. After one night in hospital, a psychiatric nurse and a junior doctor assessed that the son was not suicidal on the grounds that he said 'he was O.K.' and discharged him from hospital. Two hours later he hanged himself in the local park.

No member of staff bothered to speak to the landlord, who could have given a full account of recent problems and the fact that a suicide note had been left before he overdosed. No one bothered to contact the GP who could have told them that he had seen the patient in the past week and was treating him for severe depression. No one responded to the mother's plea to detain him.

It was amazing that the mother's concern was not one of anger or retribution, but was to ensure that such communication failure could not happen again. Subsequent detailed discussion and meetings with the hospital took place to try to introduce effective policies for communication and for proper risk assessment by experienced psychiatrists of all who present in A&E after a clear suicide attempt. Although changes to policy were made, this was only after long and detailed discussion and representation.

The mother derived some satisfaction from a devastating experience in the knowledge that her son's death may have led to a slight reduction in the probability of a similar death of another person with schizophrenia.

Issues

- Communication.
- Recognition of the superior knowledge of the relative, landlord and GP.
- The importance of adequate risk assessment.

Carers' needs

The special relationship of an informal carer to the sufferer brings with it a burden experienced by the professional carers only to a lesser extent. It is therefore all the more important to ensure that, as far as possible, carers' very real needs are met, if they are to be utilized to their most effective extent in fulfilling the needs of the person with schizophrenia, quite apart from acknowledging the needs of carers in their own right.

Empathy and understanding

Although there have been vast improvements in the past decade, carers often still come to seek advice and support only after experiencing years of rejection by the professional carers, sometimes on the grounds of 'confidentiality'. However, this alienation may lead to a sense of unwarranted despair and hopelessness and a feeling that no one understands the experiences they have had or their sense of failure to cope. Particularly in such people, the sense of belonging and sharing which can arise from contact with others who have had similar experiences gives not only relief but also an improvement in their effectiveness and sense of worth in their role as carers. The warmth and empathy which can be gained by such contacts cannot easily be given by professionals who lack this direct experience. Nevertheless, there is a minority of professionals who manage to surmount this barrier and can form such empathetic relationships with carers. More usually, even the most ardent professional believer in family involvement is viewed by carers as providing a different form of understanding and support, even if of equal importance, from that provided by support from peer groups. The two forms of support should be seen as complementary, not competitive.

The support groups and individual contact with other carers can also contribute in a variety of ways in allowing carers to come to terms with and cope with the serious problems which they face, both personal and for the person they care for.

Support

In addition to empathy and understanding, carers need more direct support in order to cope with the illness, which, especially in the early stages, will present problems that they have never experienced before. These problems will change with time and the development of the illness. Support and information systems need to keep pace with the changing requirements. More detail on the types of support needed is set out in the following sections.

Advice and information

Central to any effective support is a source of sound, reliable and relevant information and advice. Carers are often inundated with information out of context and sometimes in a vacuum. For example, it is quite unhelpful for a carer to be informed that their relative is suffering from schizophrenia, with no further enlightenment about the significance of this new information or the prognosis. In such situations, people will seek information from any source available and can be devastated by the many exceedingly negative accounts of the illness that are so abundant in the literature.

The requirements range from reliable sources of information and advice on how to get help, housing, medication and its side effects, counselling, other therapies, second medical opinions, diagnosis, prognosis, suicide, violence, effect on other family members, absconding, drugs, activities available, employment, finance, benefits, driving, genetic inheritance, the police, court procedures and the Mental Health Act.

Involvement and self-confidence

Carers, especially if they are close relatives, and more particularly so if they are parents, have often been in a position to advise the person they care for, to give them guidance or to help them in practical ways with their problems during development. They usually find that their life experiences have in no way prepared them for coping with the exigencies that arise from serious mental illness such as schizophrenia. They find that they have no knowledge of the illness and that their abilities to help and intuitive parental responses seem no longer relevant. They are often brushed aside by professional carers who assume a dominant control over the welfare of the person they care for.

There is a need to feel involved. It is gratifying to see that the benefits derived from family involvement are now being recognized and incorporated into good practice. Although much of the literature is concerned with improving family skills, some of it stresses the partnership relationship between the family, the sufferer and the professional carers (Leff et al. 1990, Smith and Birchwood 1990, Lam 1991). Slowly but surely the emphasis is shifting from seeing the family as needing treatment (Walsh 1989, Sergeant 1993) to addressing the needs of the family, including carers, and involving them in decision-making and care as an essential component of the package of care.

This change in strategic direction is reflected in recent guidance from the Department of Health (1990, 1994, 1999a) and the recent White Paper on reforming the Mental Health Act.

Only by being given a share of involvement in the formal decisions regarding care and by receiving sufficient helpful information and guidance at an appropriate time will the carer become more self-confident in addressing the needs of the sufferer.

Advocacy

Carers come from all walks of life, some of them more able than others to command attention and to get action when required. For those unaccustomed to exerting authority, it can be a daunting task to challenge professional wisdom or even inactivity, when to the carer the need for action is obvious. In such circumstances an advocate acting independently on behalf of the carer can play a useful role and can often intercede successfully on their behalf. However, it is essential that the advocate is exceedingly well informed and familiar with the system, as well as with the rights of the individual carers and sufferers and of good practice. Of course, if carers are involved, feel fully involved and their input is valued in the care of the person with schizophrenia, then the need for advocacy intervention will be diminished.

Finance: wills and trusts

At some stage many carers, especially those in their later years, will reflect on the adequacy of their provision for a mentally ill child after their death. The complicated tax laws, rules of inheritance and taxation, trusteeship and perhaps enduring power of attorney are some of the issues they will need to consider. In the case of a relative who is unable to manage their affairs because of severe mental illness, the carer may well wish to receive expert advice on the formation of suitable trusts to execute their bequests in the best interests of the sufferer. Reliable, suitably qualified and experienced legal advice is essential in these circumstances. The intricacies of mental illness are not always familiar territory to solicitors.

Even more common is a request for advice to the carer regarding the sufferer's management of their financial affairs. This is an issue fraught with difficulty. Not only is there a legal limit to the amount of family intervention permissible in such matters, but there is also the consideration of the desirability of intervening excessively in such a way as to minimize the independence of the person with mental illness. However, in many cases, especially in circumstances of acute relapse, intervention may be necessary and can sometimes be effected. The Citizens' Advice Bureau may be helpful in these circumstances. Often the more enlightened of creditors will be sympathetic and will help, when alerted to the problems. However, legal advice may often be required and the possible degree of intervention may be limited. Carers often find it difficult to accept that they can often do little or nothing to prevent a person from destroying their financial stability.

Mobility and social needs of carers

Carers need to have their own freedom to be mobile, unencumbered by the needs of the person with schizophrenia. All too often one encounters carers who feel that they must give up most or all of their own social life, sometimes even fearing to leave the house. These apprehensions are often based on the ill-founded fear of risks and the lack of carer involvement in discussions of the treatment and care of the patient. It is possible to address those needs in a non-threatening manner and in such a way that the carer comes to appreciate that there are positive benefits to be derived from making greater use of their own freedom to be mobile. Of course, in some cases, all attempts to explain the reality of the situation may fail and only in the fullness of time and with personal experience and growing self-confidence will the carer adapt to the new experience of caring for someone who is seriously ill with schizophrenia.

Respite

Carers often provide a major input to care of a person with schizophrenia. This input may range from continuous and reliable psychological support to full-time residential care in the carer's own home. Particularly in the latter case, there is a powerful need for respite. When we consider that around half of all people with schizophrenia live with families and friends in their own homes (Hatfield 1987, Department of Health 1990, Fuller Torrey 1995) it becomes obvious that a considerable part of the cost and burden of care is placed upon these informal and often unsupported carers: they are indeed a valuable and cheap resource.

It is therefore surprising that so little has been done to make respite provision for those giving continuing care at great cost to themselves. These providers of care are often by no means affluent members of society and deserve some acknowledgement of the care they give and of the burden of care they carry. Standard 6 of the National Service Framework (Department of Health 1999b) and the Carers' (Recognition & Services) Act (1995) make it a requirement for respite care needs to be assessed, but unfortunately, there is little in the way of financial support to implement the outcome.

Carers' health needs

Although the health care needs of carers are at last recognized in the National Service Framework, little is done specifically to identify these needs. Of course, most carers will attend their GP for health problems. However, there are often underlying problems arising directly or indirectly from the caring role which may not be recognized even by the carers and so may escalate before treatment or advice is sought. Perhaps the most obvious of these is anxiety, which is in part to be expected but may arise from or be exacerbated unnecessarily by lack of good guidance and information. However, it should also be remembered that because of the delayed onset and long duration of schizophrenia in most people, carers are likely to be at least middle aged and may be in their seventies or more. Little attention is given to the concomitant problems associated with old age and caring.

Often carers, especially parents, accept without question the burdens that are placed upon them, even when they are extreme and seem, to an impartial informed outsider, to be quite unreasonable. There is further information in a study by Hogman and Pearson (1995), who highlighted the special needs of carers of those with severe mental illness.

Case study – Ms G

Ms G sought help in relation to the care of her brother and the burden on her ageing parents. The mother is wheelchair bound and the father is 83. Ms G's brother has schizophrenia and is paraplegic. He returned home two months ago after a prolonged period away from the UK. The parents were informed by formal 'carers' that nothing could be done to help them. Of course, with authoritative intervention this situation was resolved.

We are clearly in a climate of change, and one could hope that such attention to the needs of carers will come as a matter of course in the not too distant future.

Support systems and access to them

Reference has been made throughout this chapter to the support systems that should be in place to support carers of people with schizophrenia. It may be useful to summarize them here and to emphasize that they must not only be available but should be utilized on a routine and regular basis. In order for this to occur it is essential that carers are made aware of them by staff at an early stage and are reminded at intervals of what is available.

Information

All carers should receive basic information about the illness, given in the form of written material and orally, preferably by the doctor. In addition they should be provided with other sources of reliable information, such as the National Schizophrenia Fellowship and MIND, as well as local organizations that are relevant. Ideally, psychiatric units should be able to provide detailed and informative reference materials at a level appropriate to the carer's needs at that time. They need good, balanced information on:

- prognosis, range of possible treatments and care
- local and national support organizations, especially support groups and groups or individuals able to give one-to-one and personal support
- treatment and side effects to be expected
- guidance on how to deal with situations that may arise.
- practice and procedures in hospital and the ward ethos
- practical information about ward visiting times, the handling of money, benefits and so on.

Guidance

While a person is in hospital, carers will need guidance on how to proceed and to cope with unexpected or unfamiliar situations. This could often be provided by well-informed and well-trained nursing staff.

Support

Carers need to be informed about support organizations that may be available. Hospital-based support groups, run by staff, provide helpful immediate sources of information and support when a sufferer is in hospital. They do not give the same type of support as can be given by carer-led support groups or by one-to-one carer support. Carers should therefore be referred at the earliest opportunity to independently run support groups, especially those run by the National Schizophrenia Fellowship and similar organizations set up specifically to cater for the needs of carers. These should be viewed as complementary to any support that can be provided by staff.

Counselling

Although the emotional needs of carers may often be fulfilled by contact with other carers in peer support groups or by individual carers, some will need professional counselling in order to cope. However, indiscriminate referrals to inappropriate or poorly qualified counsellors could be counter-productive.

Carers' rights and good practice

The Mental Health Act (1983) and Code of Practice

The Mental Health Act refers to a 'Nearest Relative', not to carers. The Nearest Relative is rigidly defined in Section 26 and cannot be varied except on the authority of the person currently given the role or by the court. There are a relatively small number of rights for carers under the Act:

- Right to require (Section 13(4)), through the local authority, an approved social worker to make an assessment under the Act. If the social worker decides not to make an application then the Nearest Relative should be informed in writing.
- Right to make an application for assessment or treatment under Section 2 or 3 respectively. However, it is considered to be good practice for the approved social worker normally to make the application, rather than the Nearest Relative.
- Right to be informed of detention for assessment or for treatment (Section 11(2)).
- Right to be consulted by the approved social worker about an application for admission under the Act (Section 11(4)).
- Right to object (Section 11(4)) to the detention of a person on Section 3. However, this right can be overturned by the Responsible Medical Officer within 72 hours (Section 23).
- Right to be informed (Section 11(3)) of the power of the Nearest Relative to discharge the patient from detention under the Act, conferred by Section 23.
- Right to be informed of discharge from detention under a Section of the Act with a period of 7 days notice, if possible (Section 133).

The Code of Practice to the Mental Health (1983) Act (published 1999) reinforces these rights.

Reforming the Mental Health Act

The White Paper, 'Reforming the Mental Health Act' (HM Government 2000) indicates that the concept of the 'Nearest Relative' is likely to be abandoned in future revision of legislation. The concept is likely to be replaced with a broader, and some would say more helpful, definition of 'carer' with rights to give and, within the limits of confidentiality, to receive, information concerning a mentally disordered person. It seems likely that many of the rights listed above are to be curtailed. However, carers are certain to be more closely involved in the future in decision-making regarding care and treatment plans and in being given vital information.

Case study: Mr and Mrs H

Mrs H has a son who lives at home with her and her present husband Mr H, but is very ill. He has repeatedly absconded from hospital and travelled all over the world. He was recently detained under Section 3 of the Mental Health Act and absconded on two occasions, while still sectioned, to the Far East and to Europe. He is clearly a survivor! Mrs H wanted to discharge her son from section but was told she is not his Nearest Relative because her ex-husband – who has little contact with him – is older.

Issues

- Mrs H was incorrectly informed of her right as the Nearest Relative.
- Was there a case for closer observation of the patient while he was compulsorily detained in hospital?

Human Rights Act 1998

The Human Rights Act came into force in English law on 2 October 2000. It reinforces the rights expressed in the European Convention on Human Rights. Most of these are already embodied in English law and the new legislation will have only minimal impact of on interpretation of the Mental Health Act since mental disorder provides one of the exceptions under which the rights of the individual may be curtailed. However, all future legislation will need to bear the Human Rights Act in mind.

Care Programme Approach

The Care Programme Approach was developed and promulgated by the Department of Health (1990). There has been a steady stream of guidance since then, culminating in *Effective Care Co-ordination in Mental Health*

Services: Modernising the Care Programme Approach (Department of Health 1999a). It contained many issues of relevance to the involvement of carers. Despite repeated circulars from the Department to health authorities, local authorities and NHS trusts, the implementation has generally been poor until recently. Even now there are still grave deficiencies in some areas. Carer involvement remains rudimentary in many places. The revised and reinforced emphasis on carers in *The National Service Framework for Mental Health* (Department of Health 1999b) and in *Effective Care Co-ordination in Mental Health Services* (Department of Health 1999a) is already leading to improvement. The new emphasis on care plans, which is emphasized even more in the White Paper on reform of the Mental Health Act (HM Government 2000), should lead to still greater improvements. Ultimately, the new monitoring, auditing and enforcing bodies that are being implemented should lead to improvement over the next decade at a pace which has so far been noticeably lacking.

The *National Service Framework*

For the first time the *National Service Framework* (Department of Health 1999b) set a series of standards in mental health. One of the seven standards is Standard 6, 'Caring about carers'. There are two main objectives which relate to 'all individuals who provide regular and substantial care for a person on CPA should:

- have an assessment of their caring, physical and mental health needs, repeated on at least an annual basis
- have their own written care plan which is given to them and implemented in discussion with them'

The framework bolsters the Carers Recognition Act of 1995, which has been poorly implemented, and *Caring about Carers* (HM Government 1999).

Role and impact of carers in treatment and recovery

The positive, or occasionally negative, impact of carers on treatment and recovery is well established (Lam 1991). Clinical intervention techniques are discussed in more detail elsewhere in this book. However, research has demonstrated that family intervention, carried out in a sensitive manner, can have a dramatic influence on the effectiveness of medication in reducing relapse (Hogarty et al. 1991). Equally, family intervention in relation to high expressed emotion is highly effective in reducing relapse rate (Leff et al. 1990).

Nevertheless, family intervention has often been reported to me by carers as 'unhelpful', 'accusatory', 'condemnatory', 'destroying family feelings' and so on. It seems clear that for family therapy to be of value, it must be carried out in a positive manner, giving support and reinforcing coping strategies, rather than finding fault or blame and giving no help with the problem, which is usually a need to reduce tension (expressed emotion) and increase ability to care. Smith and Birchwood (1990) long ago highlighted this issue and stated that

> The concept of the high EE* family has acquired an unfortunate (though no doubt unintended) pejorative connotation of the 'problem family'. It is important to remember that high expressed emotion is not necessarily in-built but arises in a complex manner from interactions between individuals of all types, including staff as well as family members, and people with a severe mental illness. Unless this is understood and acted upon, the potential benefit from family intervention can be lost.

Positive and negative aspects of clinical care

Clinical care is an essential component in the care of people with schizophrenia. At some stage, especially in the years of acute illness, periods in hospital for assessment and treatment are almost always required. Often, this in-patient clinical care provides the only available resource for reducing the destructive effect of severe relapse on the home life, social life, employment (if the person is fortunate enough to have any), relationships and all other aspects of 'normality' and normal relations which may have been built up with great effort and determination over a long period of time.

Effective intervention before such breakdowns occur should be the objective of clinical treatment. Factors that will make the intervention a positive experience for the individual and for carers will be a good outcome, a limited period of hospitalization and the in-patient experience itself. A positive clinical intervention will build upon the confidence between the clinicians, the patient and the carers, which will stand all in good stead should there be further need for intervention in the future.

Any clinical intervention should look beyond the immediate objective of terminating relapse to the longer-term objective of building up a support system to which sufferer and carer can turn with confidence and trust whenever the need arises.

Although the need for care in a hospital environment may diminish greatly with improvement in community care, there seems little prospect of

---

* EE is defined as excessive hostility, critical comments and overinvolvement of carers towards the 'ill' relative.

this in the near future. The development of crisis houses to provide short-term respite for some will probably not be the solution for those who are most severely ill, or for those whose relapse lasts for more than a brief period.

There is little doubt that medication has improved over the years. The newer 'atypical' antipsychotic drugs such as clozapine, olanzapine and queti-apine and, to a lesser extent, risperidone, seem to provide a better quality of life for those who benefit from these treatments. However, not all patients respond favourably: in some the side effects are extreme and in others there are adverse idiosyncratic responses which necessitate termination of treatment. None of the treatments represents a cure, and none is without side effects. Despite some doubts (Geddes et al. 2000, Kapur and Remington 2000) about the validity of some of the claims made for the new medications, and the suspicion that some of the reported benefits could be achieved with diminished doses of conventional antipsychotic drugs, there is little doubt that for many the outcome has been extremely favourable. Even in these cases, problems of weight gain, salivation, interference with sexual function, and sedation and lethargy persist for many.

However, there is much evidence that the value of medication is greatly increased by psychosocial interventions with the individual and with the family.

On the negative side, negative staff attitudes and behaviour towards relatives and carers 'may result in relatives becoming increasingly anxious and worried about the patient or overly protective towards them, which could lead to a decrease in the relative's effective coping' (Tarrier 1991).

Suggestions for clinicians

These suggestions summarize points made throughout this chapter:

1. View schizophrenia as an illness that affects the client and all with whom that client interacts in their life, outside hospital for most of the time.
2. Value the input and involvement from family members and other carers. Whether it is large or small, the input from those individuals may represent a large part of the social environment of your patient.
3. Understand the strains and stresses that are placed on family members and other carers when schizophrenia affects a member of the family.
4. Develop a warm, sharing and understanding, not sympathetic, attitude to clients and their carers. Sympathy may seem patronizing. Empathy deriving from experience will rarely be possible.
5. Encourage all staff to develop a positive attitude towards relatives and carers.

6. Involve the carers in consultations and decisions regarding the patient in an open, friendly, understanding and helpful atmosphere in which it is expected that all present (clinicians, client and carers) can contribute equally.
7. Emphasize the importance of equal participant input, in contrast to dominant views of clinicians. This will favour a positive outcome.
8. Involve everyone in the development of the care plan and its implementation.
9. Ensure that care plans give clear naming and means of contact with key staff and clinicians whom the patient or carer can turn to for help in times of need.
10. Ensure that regular reviews, with dates, are held for long-term patients, even when there is no immediate danger of relapse. This will help to ensure that fewer individuals will slip through the net and will foster confidence in the 'system' of care.
11. If the client is hospitalized, ensure that aftercare arrangements are conveyed to all who need to know, including the client, their carers (whether they be family members, key support workers in the community or sheltered housing), GP and any other identified individuals.
12. Ensure that an early date is set for the first review and that the date is recorded and included in the written care plan which is copied to all parties.
13. Ensure that everyone concerned feels that they have all the detailed information and support they need for the present and for contingencies.
14. If a local peer group support agency exists, encourage carers to make contact with it. If there is no such support group then encourage the development of such a group and help it to get established.
15. Ensure that family intervention techniques, such as reducing high expressed emotion, are carried out in a non-threatening manner.

References

Creer C, Wing JK (1975) Living with a schizophrenia patient. British Journal of Hospital Medicine 14: 73–82.

Department of Health (1990) Care Programme Approach. HC(90)23/LASSL(90)11; HSG(94)27.

Department of Health (1994) Guidance on the discharge of mentally disordered people and their continuing care in the community. HSG(94)27.

Department of Health (1995) Building Bridges: a guide to arrangements for inter-agency working for the care and protection of severely mentally ill people. London.

Department of Health (1999a) Effective Care Co-ordination in Mental Health Services: Modernising the Care Programme Approach. London.

Department of Health (1999b) National Service Framework for Mental Health. London.

Department of Health (2000a) New NHS Plan. London.

Department of Health (2000b) Aftercare under the Mental Health Act 1983. Health Service Circular/Local Authority Circular HSC 2000/003:LAC (2000).

Fuller Torrey E (1995) Surviving Schizophrenia, 3rd ed. Harper Collins, New York.

Geddes J, Freemantle N, Harrison P, Bebbington P (2000) Atypical antipsychotics in the treatment of schizophrenia: systematic overview and meta-regression analysis. BMJ 321: 1371–1376

Hatfield AB (1987) Families as caregivers: a historical perspective. In Families of the Mentally Ill, ed. Hatfield AB, Lefley HP. Cassell, London, pp. 3–29.

HM Government (1999) Caring about Carers: A national strategy for carers. HMSO, London.

HM Government (2000) White Paper: Reforming the Mental Health Act Stationery Office, London.

Hogarty GE, Anderson CM, Reiss DJ, Kornbith SJ, Greenwald DP, Ulrich RF, Carter M (1991) EPICS Research Group family psycho education, social skills training and maintenance chemotherapy in the aftercare treatment of schizophrenia: II. Two year effects of a controlled study on relapse and adjustment. Archives of General Psychiatry 48(4): 340–347.

Hogman G, Meier R (1995) One in Ten. National Schizophrenia Fellowship, London.

Hogman G, Pearson G (1995) The Silent Partners: the needs and experiences of people who provide informal care to people with a severe mental illness. National Schizophrenia Fellowship, London.

Kapur S, Remington G (2000) Atypical antipsychotics: patients value the lower incidence of extrapyramidal side effects. BMJ 321: 1360–1361.

Kuipers L, Bebbington P (1985) Relatives as a resource in the management of functional illness. British Journal of Psychiatry 147: 465–470.

Lam DH (1991) Psychosocial family intervention in schizophrenia. A review of empirical studies. Psychological Medicine 21(2): 423–441.

Leff J, Berkowitz R, Shavit N, Strachan A, Glass I, Vaughan C (1990). A trial of family therapy versus a relatives group for schizophrenia, two year follow up study. British Journal of Psychiatry 157(4): 571–577.

Sergeant R (1993) Schizophrenia: the problems for the family. Psychiatric Bulletin 17: 14–15.

Shepherd G, Murray A, Muijen M (1994) Relative Values. Sainsbury Centre for Mental Health, London.

Smith J, Birchwood M (1990). Relatives and patients as partners in the management of schizophrenia. British Journal of Psychiatry 156: 654–660

Social Services Inspectorate (1998) A Matter of Chance for Carers: Inspection of local authority support for carers. London.

Tarrier N (1991). Some aspects of family intervention in schizophrenia. I: Adherence to intervention programmes. British Journal of Psychiatry 159: 475–480.

Walsh J (1989). Engaging the family of the schizophrenic client. Journal of Contemporary Casework: Social Casework, February: 106–113.

CHAPTER THREE

Psychodynamic aspects of collaborative care

TREVOR JAMESON

'A powerful wizard, who wanted to destroy an entire kingdom, placed a magic potion in the well from which all the inhabitants drank. Whoever drank that water would go mad.

'The following morning, the whole population drank from the well and they all went mad, apart from the king and his family, who had a well set aside for them alone, and which the magician had not managed to poison. The king was worried and tried to control the population by issuing a series of edicts governing security and public health. The policemen and the inspectors, however, had also drunk the poisoned water and they thought the king's decisions were absurd and resolved to take no notice of them.

'When the inhabitants of the kingdom heard these decrees, they became convinced that the king had gone mad and was now giving nonsensical orders. They marched on the castle and called for his abdication.

'In despair, the king prepared to step down from the throne, but the queen stopped him, saying: 'Let us go and drink from the communal well. Then, we will be the same as them.'

'And that was what they did: the king and the queen drank the water of madness and immediately began talking nonsense. Their subjects repented at once; now that the king was displaying such wisdom, why not allow him to continue ruling the country?

'The country continued to live in peace, although its inhabitants behaved very differently from those of its neighbours. And the king was able to govern until the end of his days.'

(A traditional Sufi tale retold by Paulo Coelho, 2000, pp. 30–31)

The American Psychiatric Association's *Diagnostic and Statistical Manual of Mental Disorders* (DSM-IV) states that to make a diagnosis of schizophrenia, the patient must have been ill for at least a period of six months and has displayed at least two of the five symptom types attributed to this illness: delusions, hallucinations, disorganized speech, disorganized behaviour and negative symptoms. Also, that there is no evidence of manic or depressive symptoms, no substance misuse, or general medical conditions to which the patient's symptoms can be attributed. The overall picture is one in which the psychotic individual is out of touch with reality. Being out of touch with reality is judged by the form of the delusion, or the hallucination. A delusion is defined as the patient's belief system in one or more areas not being compatible with their culture or education, and the patient will not be persuaded otherwise. A hallucination may affect any of the five senses, leading to a falsely held perception in the absence of the appropriate sensory stimulus, the most common hallucinations being auditory or visual.

The DSM-IV goes on to tell us what to look for in the areas of disorganized speech and behaviour, and the occurrence of negative symptoms, such as a flat or blunted affect. Once a diagnosis of schizophrenia can be made we are told that the illness is to be managed by oral or intramuscular antipsychotic medication. Some acknowledgement of the side effects of such medication is made, including the possibility of tardive dyskinesia. This treatment is weighted against the debilitating effects of the illness itself.

Leuder and Thomas (2000) state that it was Pierre Janet who first formulated the concept of verbal hallucinations in his treatment of a case of hysteria, known as Marcelle, in the late nineteenth century. It was found that Marcelle would act in response to hallucinations and this led to hallucinations being viewed as impulsions and therefore, incomplete activities in themselves. For Janet, hallucinations were the direct repetitions of dissociated fixed ideas, from the patient's past experience and not always necessarily traumatic in origin or make-up. Leuder and Thomas (2000) look at the work of the pragmatists, including G.H. Mead who saw the self as the means of social control over the individual. So for Mead, voices could not be complete persons. In addressing the place of verbal hallucinations in contemporary psychiatry, Leuder and Thomas (2000) begin with a brief historical overview. They state that hallucinations are seen as pathology. Such pathology can be judged as either part of the same continuum that contains normal behaviour, or as separate (e.g. Henry Maudsley), and outside normal everyday life. The second of these views gives rise to the notion of schizophrenia as a dual personality.

In addressing the search for meaning in a person suffering from schizophrenia, Leuder and Thomas (2000) remind us that all psychic phenomena are open to endless interpretation and reinterpretation. A psychodynamic approach to schizophrenia would allow the meaningful narrative of the individual a central place in the treatment process. This approach is about the meeting of patient and therapist to engage with the patient's material, beyond the labelling of hallucinations and delusions. This is counter to the prevailing argument in psychiatry that hallucinations (and delusions) are evidence of psychosis and, as symptoms, have no inherent value or meaning. Current dogma in psychiatry would strongly recommend that any interest in the content of delusions is futile, and discussion of them should be avoided. This has taken on mythic proportions, to the extent that many clinicians believe that engaging the patient in such a manner would have the fearful and traumatic outcome of pushing that person into a far worse state of disorder. Leuder and Thomas (2000) ask the very important question, 'why are voices dangerous?' and go on to state that 'in our culture voices represent something which is to be feared' (p. 129). Instead, Leuder and Thomas (2000) produce evidence from a study to suggest that engaging with voices may be beneficial (p. 147).

One aim of administering antipsychotic medication to a person suffering from schizophrenia is to bring the delusions and hallucinations under control. In looking at the use of such medication to control verbal hallucinations, Leuder and Thomas (2000, pp.118–120) quote from a number of studies that demonstrate at least 25% of voice hearers gain little or no benefit, and may experience no reduction at all in the severity of the voices.

The defensive structure that is currently adopted by the psychiatric profession, and is pursued in its scientific knowledge base and the dominant methods of treatment employed, does much to perpetuate the split between patient and doctor: the first carrying the illness while the second holds the keys to health. Psychiatry is currently living in the shadow of its own madness. To adopt a psychodynamic approach to the treatment of schizophrenia we have to be willing to drink from the same well as the patient.

This chapter is about psychodynamic theory and how it might be used in engaging the patient on their journey. Instead of thinking about symptoms in order that they may be used to formulate a diagnosis, I consider how working within the therapeutic relationship, and addressing the contents of hallucinations and delusions, is about communication and attempts at finding meaning. It is important to differentiate between meaning for the individual and the notion of making sense. Often the lack of any 'sense' in the communication has allowed the professional to write off the patient's contribution as nonsense and therefore to be dismissed in the treatment of schizophrenia. However, meaning is about what the individual can internalize and integrate in the development of their personality. This is one of the essential tasks of any psychotherapeutic intervention in working with someone suffering from schizophrenia.

A psychodynamic understanding of schizophrenia does not have to conform to the demands of medical psychiatry: that psychopharmacology is to be the preferred intervention until more effective drugs or some form of psychosurgery replace it.

In the space allocated it would be impossible to provide a comprehensive review of the history of psychodynamic thinking in relation to schizophrenia.

Instead, I intend to concentrate on the contribution made by the depth psychologist Carl Gustav Jung. Depth psychology refers to the interest of Freud, Jung and others in the products of the unconscious. It will be important to consider some of the psychological contributions to the aetiology of schizophrenia, the development of the personality and the content of the therapeutic relationship.

I shall provide case material in order to illustrate how psychodynamic thinking can be applied in working with people who suffer from schizophrenia and in providing supervision to a variety of health professionals so that they may be enabled to extend their working practice.

Jung and schizophrenia

Jung worked as a psychiatrist at the Burgholzli mental hospital from 1900 until 1909. He was made a senior physician at the hospital in 1905 and at the same time took up the post of lecturer in psychiatry at the University of Zurich. He was to lecture on 'psychopathology, and naturally on the foundations of Freudian psychoanalysis, as well as on the psychology of primitives'. Jung was also familiar with the pioneering work of Pierre Janet on the diagnosis and treatment of hysteria. While at the Burgholzli hospital, Jung worked under Eugene Bleuler who introduced the diagnostic label of schizophrenia to replace the then current term dementia praecox.

In his essay entitled 'The psychology of dementia praecox', Jung (1907) presents a survey of some of the available views on this subject at the end of the nineteenth century and the beginning of the twentieth, and also presents insights gained from his three years of research and clinical observations based on the development of the word association test.

In concentrating on research into catatonia, Jung (1907) notes that there is a general agreement about the notion of a reduction of attention observed in the patient. The research he addresses is primarily focused on the physical effects of the disease, and Jung goes on to amplify this by suggesting that if psychic processes in catatonia are correlates of a physical series, it is not out of the ordinary as all psychic processes are correlates of all processes. Here we see ideas emerging that are to form the basis of Jung's theory of archetypes, to which we shall return later, which have both a physical and a psychic pole to them:

> What we lack is not so much comparative factual material as the way to the psychology of catatonic automatism. (Jung 1907, para. 7)

> The 'erratic' association or 'pathological idea' may therefore be a widespread psychological phenomenon which, we may at once agree with Somner, appears in its most glaring form in dementia praecox. (Jung 1907, para. 10)

Jung is already well on the way to making a case for the psychological components of schizophrenia. He goes on to investigate the work of his chief, Bleuler, looking particularly at the role of both active and passive forms of psychological negativism, and the production of active resistance. Today these would be seen as negative symptoms of schizophrenia, as defined by the DSM-IV. According to Jung (1907), Bleuler had demonstrated that negative suggestibility was not a product of the normal psyche but frequently found in the pathological symptoms of hysteria, obsessional states and dementia praecox. Jung (1907) goes on to say Bleuler observed that only a slight disturbance of feeling was needed to produce negative phenomena, e.g. reduced motor activity. This is linked to apperceptive deterioration, where the central control of the psyche is weakened and is now unable to promote positive acts, or inhibit negative ones. Jung (1907) here makes reference to the *abaissement du niveau mental*, which Janet describes in relation to obsessional states and hysteria, and its link to the deterioration observed in patients suffering from dementia praecox. Jung (1907) is able to demonstrate these symptoms by the use of his word association experiments with people suffering from hysteria, obsessional states and dementia praecox.

At the time of writing this paper, Jung had recently read Freud's *Interpretation of Dreams*, published in 1900. Freud had proposed that the dream was the 'royal road to the unconscious', portraying both a manifest and a latent content. For Jung, Freud had opened up the possibility of interpreting the meaning of dreams and a route into the unconscious that Jung was to utilize in the development of his understanding of the content of hallucinations and delusions of patients suffering from schizophrenia. For Freud and Jung, the events that take place in dreams were deemed to be of a symbolic nature and what would seem in everyday life to be bizarre needed to be interpreted. Jung later on described the language of dreams as being like that of hieroglyphics and charged us with the responsibility of cracking their coded messages in order that we might find the meaning that the dream wishes to convey to us.

In a comparison of the development and characteristics of hysteria and dementia praecox, Jung (1907) notes that the contamination that is found in word association experiments is a condensation of different ideas. He reminds us of how the same phenomenon of condensation can be found in dreams; it is through the process of what Jung called amplification that we can bring meaning to the dream. Jung (1907) remarks further on the similarity between the content of a dream and the content of an hallucination or delusion. He reminds us that every night we are subjected to the most fantastic feeling-toned experiences while asleep!

In answer to Gross's formulation that the content of consciousness is the outcome of countless unconscious psychophysical processes, Jung states

> It would seem to me more correct to assume complexes of ideas which
> become conscious successively and are constellated by previously associated
> complexes. The cement binding these complexes together is some definite
> affect. (1907, para. 56)

Further, in discussing paranoid dementia praecox he says

> Symptoms express thoughts which in consequence of their painful feeling tone
> become incompatible with ego consciousness and are therefore repressed.
> These repressions determine the nature of the delusions and hallucinations, as
> well as the general behaviour of the patient. (Jung 1907, para. 71)

Unlike Freud, Jung saw the complex as the royal road to the unconscious and
that dreams are one of the products of complexes. Jung tells us that a complex is 'the image of a certain psychic situation which is strongly accentuated
emotionally and is moreover, incompatible with the habitual attitude of consciousness' (1948, para. 201). For example, the development of a 'father
complex' would mean that any encounter that could be linked to the father
in everyday life would be highlighted in consciousness and would be accentuated. It has its own coherence and a high degree of autonomy. It can be
suppressed by consciousness with the engagement of a strong will, but only
in the short term. Jung sees the same qualities in the complexes as he
observed in the psychic disintegration found in people suffering from schizophrenia. The development of his theory of complexes led Jung to see each
individual as made up of 'many selves', and because of their autonomy, we
are not to assume the unity of consciousness or the supremacy of will.

Continuing his comparison between states of hysteria and dementia praecox Jung describes the emotional indifference found in patients suffering
from dementia praecox and how this resembles the *belle indifference* of hysteria. Jung assumes that this is due to the defensive blocking of the
complexes whereby the ideational content of affective states is diminished
and is often accompanied by excessive beliefs. He notes that explosive excite-
ments later reconfigured as traumatic events often trigger the release of such
complexes, whereby the affects are not extinguished but displaced or
blocked. In the sufferer this brings about a serious disturbance in the ego as
the complexes break through to consciousness in their very powerful
autonomous state. We observe a distinct lack of control in the behaviour and
affective state of the individual:

> A person with a strong complex thinks in terms of the complex, he dreams
> with open eyes and no longer adapts psychologically to the environment.
> (Jung 1907, para. 195)

What Jung is telling us here is that the individual is immersed in the complex to such an extent that it takes over his everyday life. In its extreme form Jung's suggestion that he 'dreams with open eyes' would denote delusory or hallucinatory behaviour. Jung (1914) tells us in his essay entitled 'The content of the psychoses' that the prevailing dogma in psychiatry is that schizophrenia is a disease of the brain. However, Jung doubts that there is any organic basis to the characteristic behaviours described as paranoia. Jung is thinking about the functional nature of this illness as denoted by Bleuler's renaming of dementia praecox as schizophrenia:

> I incline to the view that, on the basis of a disposition whose nature is at present unknown to us, an unadapted psychological function arises which may develop into a manifest mental disturbance and *secondarily* induce symptoms of organic degeneration. (Jung 1914, para. 318)

Jung (1914) accuses psychiatry of gross materialism in putting the organ of the brain above its functions, i.e. the psyche as an appendage of the brain. On looking at alterations and lesions of the brain of patients admitted to the Burgholzli mental hospital suffering from schizophrenia over a four-year period, Jung found that this accounted for only a quarter of those admitted. He concluded that this could not be a direct method of understanding psychic disturbance.

Jung (1914) noted that, from taking a number of detailed patient histories of those admitted to the hospital, the illness broke out at a time of great trauma for the individual. Jung gives the example of a cook aged 32 years who was engaged to be married. She has an anxiety attack following the extraction of teeth. She is preoccupied with thoughts that it was a sin for them to be removed and that she needed to be prayed for. Jung tells us that a biological psychiatrist would suggest that her symptoms should be regarded as those of a 'bizarre delusional characteristics of a dementia praecox'. On taking a history Jung established that she had had an affair, which had left her with an illegitimate child. The child was sent away, to be brought up in the country in an attempt to hide her shame. Of course, this meant at the time of her engagement she was racked with thoughts about what her fiancé might say if he were to discover this previous liaison. Jung tells us that she dressed up in order to impress him and this produced the first anxiety attack, as she was still preoccupied with thoughts of him leaving her. The patient displaced her shameful feelings on to her teeth. Displacement as a defence mechanism enabled this patient to express her feelings without directly facing the shame of the original cause. The problem seemed insoluble and hence the affect became overwhelming.

> When we penetrate into the human secrets of our patients, the madness discloses the system upon which it is based, and we recognise insanity to be

simply an unusual reaction to emotional problems which are in no wise foreign to ourselves. (Jung 1914, para. 339)

As with Jung's dream interpretation, he suggests once we have broken the code of psychotic communication we are able to put together the chain of events that led to the emergence of a psychotic episode, as with the example of the patient above.

Jung reminds us,

> . . . a large number of patients never find their way back from their dreams *(for some madness remains throughout their lives).* They are lost in a maze of a magic garden where the same old story is repeated again and again in a timeless present. (Jung 1914, para, 356, italics added)

Jung asks,

> Why is the mind compelled to expend itself in the elaboration of pathological nonsense? Our new method of approach gives us a clue to this difficult question. Today we can assert that the pathological ideas dominate the interests of the patient so completely because they are derived from the most important questions that occupied him when he was normal. In other words, what in insanity is now an incomprehensible jumble of symptoms was once a vital field of interest to the normal personality. (Jung 1914, para. 362)

In the transition from normal to abnormal states, the individual suffering from schizophrenia transfers elements of normal ideas into what appears to be nonsense.

In his essay on the importance of the unconscious in psychopathology given to the British Medical Association Meeting in Aberdeen in July 1914, Jung reasserts that from the viewpoint of the brain the unconscious can be seen from the perspective of both physiology and psychology. In a rather circular argument Jung states that the unconscious is the sum of all psychic events, which are not apperceived and are therefore unconscious. Those psychic events of low intensity of functioning are unable to cross the threshold from the unconscious to conscious. Jung poses the question; in what manner may we expect unconscious psychic material to behave in cases of psychosis and neurosis? For the purposes of this chapter we shall confine our interest to Jung's ideas in the case of psychosis.

Jung view is that in normal people, the principal function of the unconscious is to effect compensation and bring about balance. In acting as a compensatory agency it is akin to Freud's ideas of the dream as wish fulfilment in softening the blow of otherwise unconscious activity.

In psychosis, both in hallucinations and delusions, part of the unconscious content will force itself across the threshold of consciousness causing a loss of 'mental balance' thereby disturbing the individual's adaptation to his environment, e.g. where bizarre beliefs are held by the individual that lead him to act in a way that is not understood by others.

> The mentally unbalanced person tries to defend himself against his own unconscious, that is to say, he fights against his own compensating influences. (Jung 1919, para 457)

In this struggle the content of the unconscious that is breaking through does so in a violent manner, and the product of this is strange or alien thoughts and mood changes which are the contents of hallucinations bearing the stamp of the internal conflict. Therefore, what started out as the compensatory mechanisms of the unconscious have now broken through in ways that are totally unacceptable to conscious life.

Jung gives the following example:

> The pathological inventor, who is unable to profit by his previous failures, still allows himself, by refusing to recognise the value of his own self-criticism, to work at ever crazier schemes. He wishes to accomplish the impossible but falls instead into the absurd. After a while he notices that people talk about him, make unfavourable remarks, and even scoff at him. He believes a far-reaching conspiracy exists to frustrates his discoveries and render them objects of ridicule. By this means his unconscious brings about the same results that his self-criticisms could have achieved, but again only to the detriment of the individual, because the criticisms are projected into his surroundings. (Jung 1919, para. 460)

The distortion of these compensating influences is due to the struggle that they have against resistances to their crossing the threshold into consciousness.

In a paper read to the Royal Society of Medicine in London, Jung (1939) again addresses the nature of consciousness and the psychological causes of schizophrenia. Jung suggests that consciousness can be split into several personal consciousnesses and in normal functioning the unity of these many selves is a function of the ego complex. However, in schizophrenia the connection between the ego and some complexes is almost completely lost:

> . . . in schizophrenia the complexes have become disconnected and autonomous fragments, which either do not reintegrate back to the psychic totality, or, in the case of a remission, are unexpectedly joined together again as if nothing happened. (Jung 1939, para. 506)

It is suggested that this disassociation is often irreversible. The split-off figures do not co-operate with the conscious day-to-day life of the person suffering from schizophrenia. Jung sees this as an injury that has taken place in the personality of the sufferer to such an extent that it causes real and permanent destruction and former connections are lost. Jung suggests the scenario in which the psychotic individual has fought for many years in order to preserve his ego function and control of his personality, while the psychosis was in a 'latent state'. However, eventually he has had to submit to it in the form of strong, unconscious forces.

Central to Jung's argument is his view that

> These forces did not originate in our patient out of nowhere. They are most emphatically not the result of poisoned brain cells, but are normal constituents of our unconscious psyche. They appeared in numberless dreams, in the same or a similar form, at a time of life when seemingly nothing was wrong. *And* [my emphasis] they appear in the dreams of normal people who never get anywhere near a psychosis. (Jung 1939, para. 518)

This is a central theme; that psychosis can happen to anyone and schizophrenia is an outcome of the interplay between conscious and unconscious forces, which cause the distortion of personality and the display of certain symptom patterns in some individuals while others remain seemingly untouched by this experience. Jung would see the development of schizophrenia as something that particular individuals are disposed to because of the combination of life experiences and the make-up of their internal world. Jung (1939) suggests that dreams are the insanity of everyday life. In analysing dream material, he noted that they produced two types of character, which he called the personal character and the collective character. Further, that both these types were reflected in the symptomatology of schizophrenia, but dominated by the collective type. For Jung the collective character was made up of material from myth and legend, and the major components of these were shared across cultures. Jung (1939) charges us with the need to have a detailed knowledge of comparative psychology if we are to appreciate the contents of delusions. He tells us that schizophrenia disrupts the foundations of the psyche, producing an abundance of collective symbols, as these are the very building blocks, forming the basic structure of the personality. These symbols are generated by the archetypes.

> I call these structures *archetypes* because they function in a very similar way to the instinctual patterns of behaviour. . . . They occur in . . . the dreams, visions, and delusions of modern individuals entirely ignorant of all such 'traditions'. (Jung 1956, Early civilizations, para. 549)

Perhaps, then, it should be no surprise that the average age of onset of schizophrenia is 18–25 years, when the individual is at a most vulnerable stage of transition from childhood to adulthood.

Having moved into private practice in 1909, Jung notes the number of patients that consult him who are 'unmistakably schizophrenic' (1939, para. 539). Jung is very optimistic that the prognosis was much better for these patients because of his ability to increase their psychological understanding of the disease:

> In psychotherapy, enthusiasm is the servant of success. (Jung 1939, para. 539)

Toward the end of his life, while compiling material for his autobiography, Jung returned to the subject,

> What actually takes place inside the mentally ill? (Jung 1995, p. 135)

His assessment of the situation at the time was that although psychiatry may offer physical and more recently pharmacological containment of the patient, if only on a temporary basis, to leave the patient's inner world unanalysed was to leave the patient with little means of being able to take care of themselves in their everyday lives.

Jung (1995) tells us that it was through his work with a patient he refers to as Babette S. that he first came to understand the language of schizophrenia, which had previously been regarded as meaningless.

> More than once I have seen that even with such patients there remains in the background a personality which must be called normal. It stands looking on, so to speak. Occasionally, too, this personality – usually by way of voices or dreams – can make altogether sensible remarks and objections. It can even, when physical illness ensues, move into the foreground again and make the patient seem almost normal. (Jung 1995, p. 148)

> Through my work with patients I realized that paranoid ideas and hallucinations contain a gem of meaning. (Jung 1995, p. 148)

The content of the psyche: Jung's view of the structure of the personality

The psyche is made up of all conscious and unconscious processes. Jung saw these processes in tension, and in particular between the contents of the personal and the collective unconscious. The psyche will attempt a balancing act in order to preserve some sense of equilibrium, even as we have seen, when the collective unconscious throws up material in the form of hallucinations and delusions.

For the purposes of this chapter, we might view the structure of the personality as if in layers, one upon another, the uppermost layer being the ego. Jung viewed the ego as the centre of consciousness (Samuels, Shorter and Plaut 1986), and concerned with personal identity, but not to be confused with the sum of personality. One of the primary roles of the ego is to negotiate between the conscious and unconscious processes of the psyche, and while doing so to keep the individual focused on everyday reality. The ordering principle of the total personality (Samuels, Shorter and Plaut, 1986) is named the Self by Jung. The Self is both the centre and the circumference of the personality. In the primary state the ego and the Self are merged, but as consciousness is formed the ego begins to separate.

The layer beneath the ego is the personal unconscious, which contains the material relating to the personal experiences of the individual as well as that which has been repressed. Some aspects of the shadow are mediated by the personal unconscious. The shadow is 'the negative side of the personality, the sum of all the unpleasant qualities one wants to hide, the inferior, worthless and primitive side of man's nature, . . . , one's own dark side' (Samuels, Shorter and Plaut 1986, p. 138). The shadow is not to be confused with the mythology of split or dual personality that has been associated with schizophrenia. Instead, the shadow is archetypal and to be found in the unconscious of everyone.

The layer underneath the personal unconscious is the collective unconscious. The collective unconscious is the repository of the archetypes and is related to instinctual life. As we have already seen, it is from this deep layer of the psyche that the psychotic material of hallucinations and delusions break out, and force their way into the domain of the conscious ego.

A note on symptom relief, curing and healing

As noted above, psychotropic medication is administered in order to reduce the effects of the symptoms. Gordon (1993) reminds us that the word 'cure' comes from the Latin root *curare*, meaning to take care of, or charge of, implying a successful medical treatment. She goes on to tell us that the notion of cure is to take care of specific symptoms, and emphasizes the relationship between the carer who does something to another, the patient. On the other hand, according to Gordon (1993), healing is a process which takes account of the whole person and enables them on their journey toward wholeness. This is the process of individuation in Jungian terms. Gordon (1993) believes that the purpose of psychotherapy is to facilitate the process of healing, and that cure forms only a small part of this. For the psychotherapist must recognize that a symptom is embedded in the personality of the patient, who may well present seeking the relief of that symptom. It is the psychotherapist who must further recognize the need for work beyond the cure to enable the growth and development of the patient's psyche. Gordon (1993) would see the development of the individual who is suffering from delusions or hallucinations, as being able to 'tame' the powerful archetypal figures that are rising up from the collective unconscious. The process of individuation sees the individual engaged in the synthesis of conscious and unconscious processes. This lifelong process is the driving force behind the individual striving to reach their full potential and the accompanied search for a personal sense of meaning. A symptom would then act as a signal to the individual to pay attention to some area of the psyche in the process of individuation.

The therapeutic relationship

For psychotherapy to be effective, a close rapport is needed, so close that the doctor cannot shut his eyes to the heights and depths of human suffering. The rapport consists, after all, in a constant comparison and mutual comprehension, in the dialectical confrontation of two opposing psychic realities. If for some reason their mutual impressions do not impinge on each other, the psychotherapeutic process remains ineffective, and no change is produced. Unless both doctor and patient become a problem for each other, no solution is found. (Jung 1995, p. 166)

Case study: Robert

Robert[1] was 19 years old and in the second year of a degree course when he experienced his first breakdown. He was reading physics and had developed a keen interest in chaos theory. He found it increasingly difficult to attend lectures and this quickly came to the notice of his tutors because he had been regarded as a 'model' student. When he did attend, he found it difficult to concentrate, as he would be preoccupied by coloured patterns appearing on the walls of the lecture theatre. After a month-long struggle he returned to his parents' house and after a couple of weeks he was admitted to the local psychiatric hospital for the next five months, where he was given the diagnosis of schizophrenia and started on neuroleptic medication. During his stay in hospital, Robert continued to see these patterns and decided to keep a diary, which included his daily report of events and a drawing. When I saw the pictures Robert had made I was struck by how similar they appeared to the work of the Surrealist artist Joan Miró.

I was curious as to the meaning of these, until I came across an account by the Art Curator, Jim Ede, of his collection at Kettle's Yard, in Cambridge. When discussing a picture by Miró just inside the main entrance to the building, Ede says,

The Miró for me was an opportunity to show the students the importance of balance. If I put my finger over the spot at the top right all the rest of the

---

[1] Clinical examples are composite people and pseudonyms have been used.

picture slid into the left-hand bottom corner. If I covered the one at the bottom, horizontal lines appeared, and if somehow I could take out the tiny red spot in the middle everything flew to the edges. This gave me a much needed chance to mention God, by saying that if I had to find another name for God, I think it would be balance, for with perfect balance all would be well. (Ede 1984, p. 31)

Jung laid emphasis on the dialectical nature of the therapeutic relationship: two people meeting together in order that change may take place. Inevitably, through the therapeutic process, both therapist and patient would experience change. It is not a procedure whereby one person does something to another. Jung was eager to point out the confessional nature of the early stages of the therapeutic relationship. He saw the therapist as having taken over this role from the clergy, with the steady decline in church attendance and loss of the individual's faith in institutionalized religion. Important value is placed on the creation of a secure place, where a person can go and be accepted whatever they might need to say. This is particularly poignant in working with people suffering from schizophrenia, as often the meeting with a 'professional' is tempered by degrees of mistrust and may give rise to paranoid elements of the illness. It is important for the therapist to create a secure container for the patient, so that he may reveal his innermost secrets. Jung (1946) saw the resemblance between the developing therapeutic relationship and the alchemical process. He described the therapeutic container as the 'vas', which in alchemy is the retort where the chemicals combine. He likened the meeting between the therapist and the patient to the meeting between Adept and Soror, combining the masculine and feminine in the alchemical relationship in order to produce change. Jung (1946) represented this relationship diagrammatically as in Figure 3.1.

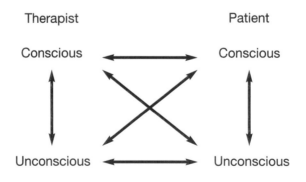

Figure 3.1 Adaptation of Jung's (1946, para. 422) diagrammatic representation of the analytic relationship.

Figure 3.1 shows the complexity of interpersonal relationships. We can see the relationship between the conscious and unconscious aspects of the therapist's psyche. The same is true for the psyche of the patient, also the interrelationship of each of these levels between the therapist's psyche and the patient's psyche.

In Figure 3.1 we can also see all possible permutations of relationship between the therapist and the patient that take place in the transference. Jung designated two types of transference relationship. First, he described the personal transference, in which the patient projected figures from their past, for example the parents, on to the therapist. The personal transference will also contain elements of the person's shadow as described above. In this relationship the therapist represents undeveloped parts of the patient's internal world. Second, he described the archetypal transference, which may contain inflated views of the therapist, for instance, believing the therapist is an omnipotent healer or the devil incarnate (Samuels, Shorter and Plaut, 1986).

Case study: Ian

Ian was barely 16 years old when he left school with no paper qualifications. He was the younger of two boys. His much older brother had left home some years ago and was in a steady relationship that had produced a baby daughter, much to the delight of both parents. After leaving school Ian drifted into a variety of jobs and youth employment training schemes, none of which he stuck at for more than a few weeks. Ian gradually withdrew from his family and his limited social life outside the family home. Instead, he took to spending long periods of time in his bedroom. He would play his music very loud, and his mother became increasingly frightened of asking him to turn it down because of the way he would stare at her with what she thought was a frightening expression of hatred on his face. Soon she would regularly hear him shouting. At first she could not make out what he was saying above the music. Eventually she could hear him angrily complaining at someone, but she knew there was no one else in the room.

Ian's mother shared her fears with his father, who was away at work in a local factory for long hours of each day. He refused to believe that there was anything wrong with Ian and instead accused him of being lazy and work shy. Ian's mother decided to call in the family doctor as Ian's behaviour persisted. The family doctor requested a domiciliary visit from a psychiatrist. The psychiatrist asked Ian to go into the local psychiatric hospital as he believed him to be suffering from a psychotic illness and that this was probably schizophrenia. Ian refused to be admitted and his mother persuaded the psychiatrist that she would do everything she could to manage her son at home. The psychiatrist gave Ian a prescription for some antipsychotic medication and agreed he would visit to review the situation. Ian did not go into hospital.

I first met Ian just before his eighteenth birthday. He had reluctantly agreed to see a therapist at the request of his mother and the local mental health team. He presented as a tall, thin young man, pleasantly dressed in casual clothes, with fairly close-cut hair. He would not make eye contact with me during the sessions for some time, except a fleeting glance where I felt he was checking my reaction to something he had said. Initially he volunteered very little information about himself or his situation. Occasionally he would grin, or laugh when there was no obvious stimulus and I thought that he was responding to a voice.

Eventually Ian told me that he would hear people passing in the street talking about him in a critical manner. While in his bedroom he would also hear the voices of the neighbours talking about him in a similar fashion. He was very surprised when I asked him what they were actually saying to him. After some time he told me some of the abusive comments they would make, often accusing him of being a little sissy who would not grow up. They would tease him about not being able to fend for himself. Ian said that when the voices got too much and he was not able to drown them out with his music, he would shout back at them in an attempt to get them to stop.

In the transference I found myself swinging between the benign mother (frightened of her son's illness and how this might manifest itself, desperately clawing him back into an inert state of childhood) and the tyrannical father (who refused to accept that his son was ill and would not grow up and be a man). I was moving between states of fragility bordering on disintegration, and omnipotent rage at the world about. I felt forced to endure these roles and survive them in order that Ian could replay these archetypal relationships over and over in the therapy, so that he could evolve into a responsible adult.

As the therapy progressed Ian was able to make a relationship with another patient of similar age he had met at the local day hospital. Ian was now able to share enough of himself with someone else in order for this relationship to evolve. They spent a lot of time together playing sport, discussing shared musical interests and visiting record shops. Ian had begun to explore adolescence more actively in his move toward adulthood.

Jung sees the process of healing in the patient as a response to the symbolic nature of the relationship, i.e. what happens in the space between the therapist and the patient. However, the psychoanalyst Harold Searles in his work with patients suffering from schizophrenia would see the therapist as initially embodying the healthy aspects of the personality, which are then reintegrated by the patient (see Sedgwick 1993). In the example of Ian above, I often found I was embodying powerful archetypal figures on his behalf and it was through my mediating these in the therapy that Ian could evolve in a new relationship to his internal world. Searles (1959) states:

> ... the inexperienced or unconsciously sadistic analyst who makes many pre-mature interpretations is thereby tending to drive the patient psychotic – tending to weaken the patient's ego rather than, in line with his conscious aim, to strengthen that ego by helping the patient gradually assimilate previously repressed material through more timely interpretations. (p. 256)

It is my experience that in the initial stages of therapy it is the job of the therapist to process the transference through either an internal or external supervisor. Interpretations should be kept to those on the way to transference interpretations and therefore not directly addressing the patient–therapist relationship. I have found that to rush in with transference interpretations can threaten the boundary of the work with patients suffering from schizophrenia, and may well lead to a situation which threatens the therapy itself. In working with Ian this was particularly so, as there were times in the work where Ian became convinced that I was colluding with the voices. When working with this type of material it is incumbent upon the therapist to be able to hold these feelings in the transference relationship, as it would be so easy to retaliate and lose the therapeutic relationship.

Case study: Robert (resumed)

Each week Robert would talk about the day-to-day events of his family life in great detail. He would repeatedly tell me the ins and outs of observations he had made about members of a family in order to demonstrate to me his ability to 'analyse' this material in such a way that I knew he was competing with me as to who might be the better therapist. When he had exhausted this material he would subject me to long theoretical descriptions of chaos theory, which – he would try to persuade me – could eventually explain everything that took place in the world. My efforts to link his material and interpret in such a way that we might go deeper, he would always manage to thwart. He would treat me as if I hadn't spoken at all and would continue with what he had to say until his line of thinking was completed. I often found myself, in these sessions with Robert, fighting to stay awake. I felt that his material was having an anaesthetic affect on me.

Searles (1959) discusses the patient–therapist relationship in the transference based on his theory that schizophrenia develops in response to a dysfunctional mother–infant dyad, which can manifest in a variety of forms. In working with Robert I was aware that he was actively trying to protect me from going crazy by his attempts to put me to sleep, and the defensive way in which he tried to close off his psychotic parts from the therapy. On reflection I am also aware that, to some extent, I was colluding with this in order to preserve the distinction between us as if Robert were the mad one and I was free of madness.

In an essay entitled 'Technique and countertransference' Fordham (1969), while paying respect to the work of Searles, describes the management of what he calls 'transference psychosis'. Fordham lays emphasis on the therapist's understanding of his countertransference as a means of guiding the therapist through the therapeutic process. He firmly believes that the therapist must retain one foot in reality. This runs counter to Jung's emphasis on the emergence of symbolic meaning and its place in the process of change. As in the example of the Sufi tale given at the beginning of this chapter, another telling of which has the Mulla Nasrudin diving into the well (the unconscious), one often finds oneself immersed in this work. This is illustrated in one's reading of Patrick McCabe's *The Butcher Boy* (McCabe 1992) where one finds oneself immersed in the psychosis of the main character before one realizes it.

Conclusion

Within the confines of this chapter I have tried to give an outline of the contribution Carl Gustav Jung made to our understanding of the psychological aspects of schizophrenia, and how this understanding has developed into a psychodynamic theory of the aetiology of the disease and its treatment. The contributions of other psychodynamic writers have been used to extend Jung's ideas, particularly in addressing the therapeutic relationship. I have purposely not engaged in an overview of psychodynamic theory in relation to schizophrenia, as this task would take us over the boundary of a single chapter.

Today the challenge is more earnest, as psychiatry moves away from the treatment of people diagnosed as suffering from schizophrenia and into risk assessment and containment. We see the momentum for this reflected in the reporting of sensationalized cases in the daily press, alongside the push for changes in legislation which will seriously undermine civil liberty.

Psychotherapy is a valuable form of treatment for patients suffering from schizophrenia, but it comes at a cost. First, the obvious financial cost of the commitment to a long-term treatment. More importantly, the cost to the patient and therapist of confronting their fears of entering into a world of madness in order that positive change might come about. This takes a toll on both participants. The therapist should not take on this work lightly, but on the basis of a full training in depth psychology, detailed knowledge of working with schizophrenia and appropriate supervision. A depth psychotherapy training takes at least four years to complete and includes personal analysis (minimum three times weekly) throughout the length of the training; four years of theoretical seminars; clinical seminars (for a minimum of three years); the supervised treatment of patients (one male and one female for a minimum of three times weekly each over two years); a period of infant observation and a psychiatric placement. This training should always be undertaken with a registered body such as the UK Council for Psychotherapy (UKCP) or the British Confederation of Psychotherapists (BCP).

Increasingly research is being published (see Martindale et al. 2000) demonstrating the efficacy of psychotherapeutic treatment for schizophrenia over a period of two years or more. While the myth of science moves ever onwards, psychiatry awaits a chemical cure for schizophrenia, but Hauke (2000) challenges us:

> To what extent are we, just as the Victorians with their 'savages', reading the semiotics of psychosis as merely full of error – to be cured partly by education, but mostly by chemical correction? (p. 270)

References

Papers by Jung that appear in his collected works are from the edition published by Routledge and Kegan Paul, translated from the German by R.F.C. Hull, edited by Sir Herbert Read, Michael Fordham and Gerhard Adler. The reference will give the name of the paper and the volume of the collected works.

Coelho P (2000) Veronika Decides to Die. HarperCollins, London.
Ede J (1984) Kettle's Yard: A way of life. Cambridge University Press, Cambridge.
Fordham M (1969) Technique and counter-transference. In: Fordham M, Gordon R, Hubback J, Lambert K. (eds.) (1989). Technique in Jungian Analysis, 2nd edn. Karnac Books, London.
Gordon R (1993) Bridges: Metaphor for psychic processes. Karnac Books, London.
Hauke C (2000) Jung and the Postmodern: The interpretation of realities. Routledge, London.
Jung CG (1907) The psychology of dementia praecox. Collected Works, Volume 3.
Jung CG (1914) The content of the psychoses. Collected Works, Volume 3.
Jung CG (1919). On the problem of psychogenesis in mental disease. Collected Works, Volume 3.
Jung CG (1939) On the psychogenesis of schizophrenia. Collected Works, Volume 3.

Jung CG (1946) The psychology of the transference. Collected Works, Volume 16, 2nd edn.

Jung CG (1948) A review of complex theory. Collected Works, Volume 8, 2nd edn.

Jung CG (1956) Recent thoughts on schizophrenia. Collected Works, Volume 3.

Jung CG (1995) Memories, Dreams, Reflections. Fontana, London.

Leuder I, Thomas P (2000) Voices of Reason, Voices of Insanity: Studies of verbal hallucinations. Routledge, London.

Martindale B, Bateman A, Crowe M, Margison F (2000) Psychosis: Psychological Approaches and Their Effectiveness. Gaskell, London.

McCabe P (1992) The Butcher Boy. Picador, London.

Samuels A, Shorter B, Plaut F (1986) A Critical Dictionary of Jungian Analysis. Routledge and Kegan Paul, London.

Searles HF (1959) The effort to drive the other person crazy – an element in the aetiology and psychotherapy of schizophrenia. In: Searles HF (1986). Collected Papers on Schizophrenia and Related Subjects. Maresfield Library, London.

Sedgwick, D. (1993). Jung and Searles. Routledge, London.

CHAPTER FOUR

Schizophrenia and occupational therapy

SALLY GOLDSPINK AND SARAH NEWMAN

Occupational therapy and its antecedents

History of the profession

Occupational therapy is a relatively young profession, but its guiding principles are many centuries old: Galen (130–200 CE) suggested 'employment is nature's best physician and essential to happiness' and encouraged digging, fishing and house-building (cited in Macdonald 1970, Turner 1974). By the early twentieth century the notion of activity in the treatment of mental illness had become commonplace. At this time the views and ideas that made up the fabric of society were changing. Women were leaving the confines of the home and were taking up 'respectable' occupations. It was in this climate that Dr Elizabeth Casson pioneered the first school of occupational therapy in 1930, and most of the recruits to the profession, then and since, have been female. The profession soon became formalized, with the formation of the English Association of Occupational Therapists in 1936.

The role of occupational therapy came to the fore with the treatment of servicemen disabled during the Second World War. This led to the development of the World Federation of Occupational Therapists in 1951 and, in the UK, State Registration in accordance with the Professions Supplementary to Medicine Act (1960) as described in Turner (1974).

What is occupational therapy?

Occupation describes a range of activities from employment, to swimming, to listening to music – it is 'doing something', filling our time. The notion of 'occupation' is considered in all areas of social sciences, including philosophy and sociology. To have attracted such attention, 'doing something' must be important.

Occupational therapists are viewed by other professional colleagues and clients as the people who fill time, provide activities and make sure people can cook, but principally these are by-products of what occupational therapists are really interested in. Their primary interest lies in the connection between the individual, their environment and the subsequent impact on their everyday ability to function (Creek 1992).

When the question is rephrased as, 'What do occupational therapists do?' we enter a whole new arena. Occupational therapy is constantly striving to define and redefine itself. Chevalier (1997, p. 539), speaking of the *Journal of Occupational Therapy*, states 'compared with any other medical or paramedical journal, this degree of philosophical speculation or soul-searching is extraordinary'. Occupational therapy is about people; it places emphasis on volition. This means that there may never be one single answer to 'What do occupational therapists do?'

Meyer (1977) suggested that occupational therapy centred around providing opportunities as opposed to 'prescribing activity' within the parameters of an individual's interests and culture. Mayers (2000) translates this view into a three-point summary of occupational therapy:

• Meaningful activity (occupation) is the core to intervention.
• Activity must be balanced to include all areas of an individual's life.
• Opportunities for activity must enhance problem-solving and planning in order to enable ownership of decisions.

This means that there is no place here for simply 'giving somebody something to do'. People cannot be simply slotted into activity; the activity itself must be moulded and shaped to the individual's intrinsic needs.

Gender inequalities in occupational therapy

Given its historical roots, and the fact that over 90% of occupational therapists are female (Brown 1998, cited in Pollard and Walsh 2000), it is little wonder that the stereotypical female role and all that goes along with it are seen by other professions as the components of 'occupational therapy'. Knowledge, when institutionalized and controlled through education and training, has played a central role in maintaining gender inequalities and confusion about this approach to therapy. Indeed, Keddy et al (1986) go as far as to suggest that the problem with professional identity and definition for occupational therapy is simple:

occupational therapy = female vocation
female vocation = domestic chores.

Today, however, people within our society – male and female – are spending less and less time engaged in domestic chores. Labour-saving devices have taken much of the hard work out of domestic life, but this has not been reflected in the stereotype of occupational therapy. This clearly demonstrates the point Fair (1999) makes when suggesting that there is an implied 'correct' method for activities of daily living and goes on to argue that there is little to be gained for individuals from engaging in unfamiliar functional activities, utilizing unfamiliar methods and which, generally, have little meaning to them.

Something to do

Occupation in the traditional mental asylum

Murphy (1991, p. 38) describes the regime in the traditional mental asylum as 'sleep, work, eat, sleep' and Barham (1992, p. 36) equated the asylum to a small town:

> The traditional hospitals were spacious, within equally spacious grounds, providing occupational and industrial therapy, art, music and pottery, dieticians, religious studies, organised outings, libraries, patients clubs, subsidised boutiques and friendship networks established over many years.

People with schizophrenia were given a life, given things to do, their time was filled for them. Individuality, choice and the right to say no became the price of having something to do. 'Wellness' was measured by compliance . . . sounds familiar?

Compliance

Compliance means many things, but for the purposes of this work it relates solely to whether clients are doing what we, the professionals, think they should be doing. However, the tide is turning. There is a growing impetus to look at compliance differently. Gamble and Brennan (2000) identify very real reasons for non-compliance in our service users. Could it be that they are so sedated by medication that they are physically unable to go to the day centre or outpatient appointment, or possibly that their loss of volition and motivation is such that they do not attend (Heyward, Kemp and David 2000)? Before clients are labelled 'non-compliant', we as professionals should re-assess what we are doing and our expectations of our clients. This can only be done using standardized and validated assessment tools with the clients, and engaging them by doing so. Fowler, Kuipers and Garety (1995) suggest that the engagement process of any therapeutic relationship is 75 per cent of the work.

As professionals perhaps we need to change our approach, and allow service users to have control, information and understanding about their illness, service provision, and why we do what we do.

The need for 'doing'

'Why do we do the things we do?' is a simple but powerful question that applies to all aspects of life. This question makes us examine our purpose, our role, our place in life; it makes us wonder what we would be doing if we didn't do the things we do; it makes us smile at some of the things we do and feel sad at others.

So, why do we do the job we do? It is often considered that individuals reflect their own personal needs, values and interest through their chosen profession. Other intrinsic factors include the promotion of self-worth, the respect and recognition of a 'job well done'. Jahoda (1981) places emphasis on the social role given to us because of the job we do. Roles adapted via our work provide us with identities within our community and the perceived social position, morality and trustworthiness associated with it. Society, in the broader sense, and the community in the more local sense, have rules and expectations of all the members who live within it. This is governed to some extent by laws of the land; nevertheless, having a job, whatever that job may be, allows the community in which we live to define expectations and make assumptions about us. What is at stake in the issue of public image is the capacity that an occupation has to ground its claims for professionalism in the public acceptance of its knowledge and skills. Public image remains important. These images can be used in a number of ways – to influence powerful groups (such as politicians), funding and training – but these images are interwoven with the self-images of professionals. The public contain the clientele, and the clientele provides a mirror for the maintenance of occupational identity (Hugman 1991).

Argyle (1985) suggests that job satisfaction can be measured in many ways, but to some extent is very personal. He also suggests that the job that we do is not that important, but the satisfaction, happiness and sense of achievement it may bring are. Paloutzian and Ellison (1982) suggest that satisfaction with occupation, however small, relates to 'existential well-being'. For example, if we feel valued, our occupation has a purpose and we have an idea of where that might lead, then satisfaction occurs.

Ornstein and Carsten (1991) put forward the idea that from early childhood we in the Western world are bombarded with occupational expectations: 'What are you going to do when you grow up?', 'Will you follow in your father's footsteps?', 'You need to work hard at school, people with degrees are more likely to get a good job', and so on. There is no mention of life events that could have a negative impact on these social aspirations. What parents would say to their child, 'Enjoy the dream of your chosen career, because one person in 100 develops schizophrenia, and your life, your sense of individuality, choice and freedom may stop when you reach 17'?

But why does the world of psychiatry deny people who have schizophrenia the same right to ask 'Why do I do the things I do? Maybe it's just too difficult, perhaps this would open the door for professionals to examine their own occupational identities, too intertwined with their self-identities. Psychological bonds with work enable us as citizens to consider ourselves as having careers or vocations as opposed to just 'having something to do' (Rathus and Nevid 1989). The work gives us an identity.

Perhaps this is why the painful acknowledgement of a severe and enduring mental illness is what professionals strive to avoid facing; we try to mask the true experience by continuing to give people 'things to do'.

Problems for mentally ill people

Turner and Ten Hoor (1986) discuss six global issues associated with people who have schizophrenia:

- problems with rudimentary activities of daily living
- difficulties in consistently obtaining food, shelter and clothing
- perceived deficits in their motivation/accessing services
- exceptional sensitivity to stress
- overt and covert behaviour that inhibits or acts against their own sense of well-being or that of others
- an illness that cannot be treated by short-term, single-mode treatments.

Along with these six factors, all of which are directly related to the individual's presenting mental state, social stigma remains a major stumbling block. Maybe it is this stigma that we professionals, as members of the same community as the mentally ill, must associate with.

Because of the nature of the illness and the symptoms presented, the lifestyles of those with schizophrenia are misunderstood. As professionals we often make assumptions about the 'symptoms' presented to us, but sometimes what we see is not how it really is for the client. Hinshelwood (1999) reminds us that hallucinations and delusions are entirely personal and idiosyncratic, so it is important to engage and get to know the client before implementing a care package. Fowler, Kuipers and Garety (1995) suggest that a useful way to investigate this further is to use the so-called 'Columbo technique' of questioning. (One of Detective Columbo's trademarks was that he would start to leave and when he was almost out the door he would stop and say, 'Oh. Just one more thing' – which was the really important one.)

The devil finds work for idle hands

For many mentally ill people, employment and the aspirations and demands associated with it become a mountain too high to climb. In the present social climate, the prospect of unemployment looms. This of course means time to fill, and potentially lots of it.

For many of us, what would be the alternative to working? Parsons (1952) goes as far as suggesting that many of us fear 'idleness', because without work, we would feel lost, useless or bored, or 'go crazy' with the prospect of too much time on our hands. But would we have time on our hands, or would we spend more time doing the things we want to do, such as walking, exercise, baking, painting, learning a new language? Without work, we might not know what to do with ourselves. Work or 'doing something' makes us turn our attention outwards; idleness would confront us with ourselves, which might be intolerable. So would we really be idle, or would we be just changing our views of what work is? Work has become the bedrock of our identity and success, but the evolving world of work has become unstable. We now build our lives on a precarious situation, like skating on thin ice. External realities and routines mean that we have no time or space to indulge in nightmares, dreams or fantasies. Therefore, by allowing those with schizophrenia too much free time, we condemn them to themselves, a prospect 'well' people strive to avoid.

Expectations

We all have expectations of ourselves, our family, our friends, our colleagues and our clients; but where do they come from? And what defines them? How can one person's expectations be so radically different from someone else's? Perhaps the answers lie in 'experience', culture and social backgrounds.

How many times in our working lives have we heard 'I expect he won't turn up' or 'I expect he is still in bed'? When we work in such close proximity to our clients' lives, and when we are faced with the knowledge that potentially we know everything about a person's life, and we actually know nothing about them as a person, it becomes easy to play the expectation card. Do we as professionals really have the right to expect anything of our clients? Perhaps the expectation should be turned on us: 'I expect my health-care professional to turn up on time'.

In order to fully appreciate society's expectations of someone with schizophrenia, we must take into account some of the varying symptoms they experience and the problems these lead to.

Do expectations cause disability? Ekdawi and Conning (1994) assert that when a person's problems are accommodated for they are no longer

Case study: Mr A

Mr A is 23 years old and lives alone in a council flat. He has been unemployed for five years. After leaving school with five GCSEs he began but did not complete an information technology course. At present he is not in a relationship. He does not get on well with his family and has only a few friends. He occasionally smokes cannabis, and spends most of his day in bed because he watches television most of the night.

What are the expectations on Mr A? As long as he abides by the law, complies with the requirements of the benefits agency/job centre and abides by his tenancy agreement, he meets society's basic expectations.

Now consider the situation again with the additional information that this man was diagnosed with paranoid schizophrenia five years ago. He has had four admissions to hospital, three of which were under the Mental Health Act, is overweight and is currently on intramuscular depot medication weekly, takes antidepressants and anticholinergic medication.

What are the expectations now (in addition to the three previously mentioned)?

- to attend regular consultant psychiatrist appointments
- to accept depot medication weekly
- to alert his CPN immediately if he experiences any paranoid thoughts
- to collect repeat prescriptions from his GP
- to collect his medication from the pharmacy
- to inform health care workers of all aspects of his life.
- to comply and participate in a care plan for a support worker
- to comply with adequate diet, exercise and health promotion advice
- not to use cannabis
- to attend dietician appointments and comply with advice
- to ensure the flat is clean and tidy and allow his CPN to assess it weekly
- to collect his benefits from the Post Office weekly
- to budget his money
- to look clean and tidy
- to get out of bed every morning
- to leave his flat daily
- to attend a social skills group once a week
- to develop a relationship with his family
- to comply with efforts to improve and maintain his social networks.

disabled, it is the environment that disables. For example, if a deaf person successfully uses a hearing aid, are they still disabled?

Waxler (1977) considers that specific illnesses and disabilities are relatively defined according to the society in which they are found. Once defined, society and therefore cultural cues indicate given roles. Marsella (1988, cited in Sullivan 1994) exemplifies how culture influences an individual's experience and interpretation of disability given the social response they receive.

Warner (1983, cited in Sullivan 1994), compares how there is far more room for recovery in the developing world because of the differing nature of 'expectation' and the concept of recovery as a 'community phenomenon', as against the community segregation of Western institutionalization.

Anthony (1977, as cited by Ekdawi and Conning 1994) describes how rehabilitation needs to include physical, intellectual and emotional abilities to live with only the smallest degree of support from mental health services. This view has been substantiated by Ross (1993), who acknowledges the risk of day centres transforming themselves into 'psychiatric ghettos' and working directly against people utilizing resources within their own community.

So why can't we work with our clients in their community in the way that they want us to? Is it because it again leaves us as professionals exposed to our own inadequacies, idiosyncrasies and inabilities, or is it to do with who has control and power? Surely we cannot show our clients that we are anything other than perfect. As professionals (of any discipline) we must not forget that we are not immune to the social stereotypes and expectations that we are raised with. Where does that leave us in the area of modern community work?

Assessment

We tend to view our clients' lives as little boxes that we, the professionals, dip in and out of from time to time without really understanding what the boxes are made of, what's in them, or how one is related to another. Abdullah (1995) argues that in order to achieve a holistic approach to the individual, their culture, beliefs and traditions must be considered and understood. This is also discussed by Birchwood and Tarrier (1994), Fowler, Kuipers and Garety (1995), Chadwick, Birchwood and Trower (1996) and Garety, Fowler and Kuipers (2000), who suggest that a process of engagement is required. This should be followed by a thorough assessment.

But who assesses what? Hugman (1991) suggests that so many professionals now lay claim to the same practices – risk assessment, counselling, management of resources, and rehabilitation – it is becoming unclear exactly which profession does what. The ability to work together with other professions is important, but the obstacle most health care professionals perceive as obstructive is the medical profession. Hugman (1991) suggests that health care professionals struggle with this, as it is seen to prevent their occupational autonomy. The ambiguous relationships between professions can cause occupational confusion.

There has been a gradual emphasis on separate assessments being made by the various therapists (Mocellin 1988). This can often be interpreted by the medical profession as a threat, and attempts are made to redefine caring professionals back to the periphery of medicine, and thus maintain them in a subordinate role (Wallis 1987) rather than facilitating skill mix, professional innovation and creative care planning (NICE 2002).

Intervention

Before any intervention is considered, two key concepts must be acknowledged: motivation and meaningful occupation. Mayers (2000) asserts that clients have the knowledge of what they want, their own personal assets and their own ideas of meaningful activity, so why do professionals overlook the obvious? Why don't we just ask the clients? Could it be that we as professionals may be uncomfortable with the answer we receive? And what happens if we disagree with the answer? After all, who really are the experts?

Ekdawi and Conning (1994) discuss how we might attribute 'labels' to our clients when they do not 'perform' to our professional expectations (or rather, when they do not do what we want them to). When the hours of skill development or personal management appear to have made little difference, surely we need to ask ourselves why. Has the situation been accurately assessed, and is the intervention really needed? Could we be doing something differently, more beneficial – and if so, what? Clients become tarnished with the 'lacking in motivation' tag or 'is this negative symptomatology or is he just lazy' as differential diagnosis. What if the real reason, the most obvious reason, the reason which is always overlooked (because it can't be possibly be true – we know best) is simply that we have not connected with that client, we have not understood his pain, his difficulty, his needs. We have simply placed our bag of expectations on his shoulders and walked away.

Sullivan (1994) describes 'rehabilitation' in terms of social role, cutting through the perceived stereotypes and focusing on interventions that lessen or even eliminate the social disability that comes with severe and enduring mental illness by acknowledging and enhancing self-worth and esteem. The paradox is that these people remain 'our clients'. Professionals pay a great deal of attention to improving their clients' confidence, developing techniques of assertiveness, only to be baffled when a client opens the door and says 'No, I don't want to see you today'. Automatically, the professional expectation kicks in: 'My patient is unwell'. Have we not just spent weeks encouraging and supporting this client to do this? Why the surprise? Surely it is safer for them to test it out on us first. Do we allow our clients ever to be well? Is this because we, the professionals (by virtue of the illness model) expect them not to be well?

The dilemma is beautifully illustrated by a 'communication group': once the professional arrived to lead the group, the spontaneous chatting and conversation stopped in readiness for the lesson on communication.

The perceptions an individual elicits *from* others are likely to have significant implications for the way they are treated *by* others (Trower et al. 1978). For instance, someone who is experiencing paranoid ideas may refuse to interact with others, which may in turn lead these others (e.g. professionals) to consider the person to be moody or aloof, which in turn leads to negative non-verbal cues, thus reinforcing the paranoia (Argyle 1983).

Role and public image

There is no getting away from the fact that we are all defined by our roles: 'parent', 'partner', 'patient', 'professional'. We are all 'assessed' in some way or other, by the way we dress, a 'bad hair day', the state of the home we live in; it's just the outcomes that are different, the reasons that others read into our actions, the answers to 'why do we do what we do?', the overall degree of importance that any situation or interaction is given.

What is at stake in the issue of public image is the capacity that an occupation has to ground its claims for professionalism in the public acceptance of its knowledge and skills. Public images remain important. Image is interwoven with self-images of professionals. The public contain the clientele, and they provide a mirror for the maintenance of occupational activity (Williams et al. 1987). It is part of the professional ideology, usually expressed as an ethic of service, that the professions exist for the benefit of any member of society who has need of their expertise. However, there has been a long crescendo of critical opinion which argues that such claims meet the needs of the professions rather than those of service users (Wilding 1982). Hugman (1991) goes on to suggest that the critical perspective implies that professions seek to control patients or clients not only by exercising power over them, but also to the extent of defining who and what a client is and should be, thus defining their 'care'.

Hugman's use of the term 'client' and 'patient' is a deliberate one. It implies a number of things:

- Becoming a client or patient conveys roles of socially constructed objects of professional power.
- Nurses, social workers and occupational therapists have their patients defined for them by doctors.

- The presumption is that these people 'must' be helped, irrespective of whether or not they want to be helped.

All professionals have considerable power over potential clients, through knowledge of diagnosis, how 'the system works' and the rules that are applied (Rickman and Goldthorpe 1977). Becker (1970) suggests that classification and terms used in relation to patients are based on the problems that the service users pose for the professionals in achieving their occupational goals.

Direct and indirect forms of control are imposed on our clients. Professionals can coerce, contain and direct the patient, imposing control; but what happens if the patient refuses or resists? Are they really being 'difficult'? Hugman (1991) suggests that in the context of the 'caring' services, this control can include all aspects of a person's life. Where someone lives, with whom they live, the work they do, the education or leisure pursuits they undertake, the food they eat, whether and where they smoke, the clothes they wear and their access to and use of money may all be under professional supervision, with varying degrees of subtlety. Day (1981) identifies that the compliance of the client can be sought through the threat of a more coercive outcome.

Clearly, the more desirable areas of work are those that allow the professional scope to practice virtuoso skills, and the 'good' client is the one whose problems permit the professional to practise these skills in a way that is valued professionally. The 'good' client accepts the professional's methods of working, including the definition of needs and goals.

The 'bad' patient is one who attempts to assert their own demands, to subvert or exploit the professional's intervention (Pithouse 1987). Such a client may be seen as difficult, non-compliant, manipulative, or even 'personality disordered'. Certainly, there is no denying that these clients can be hard work, but this is our problem, not theirs, and surely it is therefore our responsibility to work together to offer the help they feel is required. Satyamurti (1981) offers an explanation for this: the ascription of responsibility serves to undermine the standing of the service user as a capable person and promote the generalization that people who need the caring services are incompetent. He goes on to suggest that professionals maintain social distance from their clients and says that this is a response to a fear of being controlled by the service user. This can be exemplified by the use of separate toilets, doors marked 'staff only', and the general formality of interaction found in day centres and hospital facilities. For example, instead of the sister of a ward introducing herself as Jane Jones, she will often introduce herself as 'I am the charge nurse, Sister Jane Jones.' The assumption is that Jane Jones' title defines her role, and reflects that she has status and the patient does not. Thus the patient is in a position of possession by the professional, and is at a distinct disadvantage, knowing nothing about the charge nurse, yet she, before even meeting the patient, knows a lot of information about them.

The distance maintained between caring professionals and their clients is itself part of the stigmatizing process. Maintaining social distance not only provides the professional with power, it also serves to sustain the self-image of the professional. It reinforces the commonsense notions of nurses and occupational therapists as competent and caring. To the extent that 'our' clients are incompetent, 'our' competence is reinforced – we are capable when they are not (Dingwall 1977).

What changes are needed?

We need to consider dramatic changes in approach, thinking and training. There is not a single set of uniform expectations for each profession and so there is inter-professionally disputed territory (Keddy et al. 1986).

To presume that our every move is under scrutiny is somewhat unnerving, but isn't that what we subject our clients to, with the unconditional requirement that they accept it? We should therefore take a more global view of our clients over a long period of time. Why should service users accept all of this?

As professionals we set ourselves apart from our clients: the phrase 'what's good for the goose ...' is somehow not applicable here. To presume that we all have the same reactions, coping strategies and difficulties is preposterous, so what are social skills groups all about? Can a group setting really address the individual nature of social circumstance? Surely the individualistic nature of social functioning makes it impossible to provide a 'general prescription' for success?

Skills in society

When someone is diagnosed with severe and enduring mental illness the perceived notion is that they become askilled (lacking in skill) in every area of their life. It is as if arriving on 'Planet Mental Health' means that any previously attained (and probably maintained) skill no longer exists. We, the professionals, suddenly need to set up cooking groups and to ensure individuals are equipped to 'maintain their environment' (which means make their beds). However, the ability to transfer skills (e.g. from a ward kitchen to the home environment) is limited (Allen 1992). So is it that these clients need to cook, or that we need to give them something to do? Or should we really be looking at the reasons behind why they do not prepare food for themselves? Could it be that it is too stressful, their symptoms are too distressing, or the side effects from their medication prevent them from doing so?

The simple fact is that people no longer need to be able to 'cook' in the traditional sense. The vast array of food available in our supermarkets and high streets – convenience foods, takeaways, ready meals – means that life in the kitchen does not have to be time-consuming or difficult for anyone any more. Ekdawi and Conning (1994) cites a story of a man with a long history with psychiatric services who lived alone in the community. He was assessed to have problems with cooking and so was provided with a programme to teach him to cook. As time went on he was visited again for a progress review, to the dismay of the occupational therapist who found no shred of evidence to suggest any cooking activity. When asked why his new cooking skills had not been implemented, the man replied that for many years he had enjoyed his evening meal with his friends in a local cafe!

We work in a safety-conscious culture. We perceive the level of danger experienced by our clients in their everyday activities to be of paramount importance – the likelihood of distraction while frying a pan of chips, the potential dangers of smoking in the kitchen. Of course there is no denying that these risks exist, but they exist for everyone. What we really need to be asking is how our client's current mental state impacts on their daily life, not simply questioning their level of safety in the kitchen. It's the reasons why they might be unsafe that are important.

We are also far too concerned about everyone having a 'healthy diet', which is great if you have the requisite skills and finances to do this. Surely, rather, we need to support these clients in doing what they can and recognizing the skill involved. Consider deciding to have fish and chips for tea. This may seem a simple procedure on the surface, but it involves many small tasks:

- Have I got enough money?
- How do I get there?
- Are they open?
- What sort of fish would I like?
- Remember to take house keys with me

and so on. Our clients don't starve themselves because they can't cook; perhaps they go without because they are so distressed by their mental state. So, where does the work really need to be done?

Abdullah (1995) describes the void that exists between patients and professionals when considering areas of 'patient need'. Who decides, and what are the decisions based on?

Domestic chores and other activities of daily living need to be considered in the context of the effects of institutionalization and the high incidence of schizophrenia among young men, which may mean that the transition from family dependence to personal independence is grossly skewed. However, once again, expectations need to be based on today's society and in conjunction with the expectations of patients and their peers. Dusting the bedroom is not central to the life of an 18-year-old. Boyle and Andrews (1992) confirm the need to ensure that services consistently provide care that is both relevant and acceptable to the individual.

The concept of independence

A common word used in mental health work is 'independence', as in 'your care plan is devised to increase your level of independence'. It's as if 'independence' is the cornerstone departments are built on. We never see it, or examine it, we simply have faith that it is there. What does 'independence' actually mean? The dictionary refers to it as; 'not subject to others, self-reliant, free'. Can we say that this definition reflects our lives? Are any of us 'not subject to others'? Indeed, in our society is it even possible to consider a life that is not 'subject to others'? Is this what we are really striving for in the work with our clients? Do we give them a map for their journey, knowing that they will never reach their destination? It may be argued that this one ideal separates professions. Does the road to independence take us in different directions to experience different journeys to reach the same mythical destination?

The conflict in professional terms could be in the varying opinions and speculation attributed to the understanding of action and activity as a means to independence, with the added irony that in a culture which values 'independence' so highly, the internal and external pressures placed on the person with schizophrenia mean greater expression of the illness. Striving for 'independence' may actually make people more dependent.

Case study: Mr A (resumed)

Let's assume that Mr A does not get out of bed one day. It would be simple to note another Did Not Attend in a Cardex file and miss the many potential reasons for this:

- Is he too scared to get up?
- Are his voices telling him not to get up?
- Is he unable to sequence actions to get up?
- Is he experiencing side effects of his medication?
- Is he tired because he stayed up to watch a late movie?
- Is his flat too cold?
- Does he want to be left alone today?
- Does he not want to go swimming with his support worker?
- Does he have anything to get up for?
- Does he enjoy being in his comfortable bed?

Allen (1992) focuses us on the idea that it's not what people say, it's what they do that provides specific interest to occupational therapy. In our everyday working lives it becomes easy to overlook what our clients are trying to express through what they do, as exemplified by Mr A's behaviour. Crabtree (1998) concludes that is not difficult to become 'seduced by language'. Speech is given preference to action. Allen (1992) concurs with this idea and puts forward the necessity of re-evaluating activity and perceptions of activity to emphasize the fact that it's not that people won't do things, it's that they can't. For some reason, they are unable to fulfil the expectations that they put on themselves or are put on them by others.

Occupational therapy (unlike other professions) is adept in compensatory interventions. Difficult, meaningless or impossible tasks can be compensated for to make space for meaningful, achievable activities. We all make our lives easier in this way, each time we turn on the dishwasher, get in a car, or buy bread from the supermarket. Allen (1992) remarks 'the motto "no pain, no gain" is not recommended'. It may sound obvious, but it's putting into practice the idea of accepting people for who they are.

> Humans make meaning of their lives despite their dependence or lack of function and despite sometimes cruel social circumstances and inhospitable environments. (Crabtree 1998, p. 207)

Collaborative working

For the purposes of this chapter, collaborative working means two things: one is the area of working collaboratively with the clients and the other is working collaboratively with other professions.

We should take time to engage with service users, and during this time we should begin to assess and engage with our clients. This process may take up to two years of weekly one-hour sessions (Kingdon and Turkington 1991, Fowler, Kuipers and Garety 1995). Chadwick, Birchwood and Trower (1996) emphasize that this approach affords the client both power and empowerment, whereas the medical model offers the client no autonomy or control over their care and treatment. The idea that we engage clients in areas that they want to work on may seem very alien, and contradictory at times, but surely it is the most sensible and obvious approach to take.

Case study: Mr B

Mr B is 28 years old. He has a diagnosis of schizophrenia, and has had contact with the mental health services since he was 15. He denies he is mentally ill, but has a florid psychosis based around religion and believing that he is the chosen second Messiah. He says that his main problem is 'emptdepression'. He is cautious of the services as he reports that nobody has ever listened to him or believed him, and says that when he does tell community workers about himself and his beliefs, they get him sectioned and taken into hospital.

How do we engage this man? We talk with him about his 'emptdepression', which he can describe in detail as having an empty mind and feeling low in mood. This leads on to him discussing how he manages when he feels like this. As a result we discovered over a period of 12 months that this man dealt with his low mood by binging (several loaves of bread, four packets of Mr Kipling cakes, two family packs of biscuits, chocolate bars, six packets of crisps – all in one sitting). He would then feel guilty because he would not reach his target weight of 10 stone (the weight that he thought Jesus was on the cross) and so would vomit and exercise furiously.

By allowing Mr B to discuss what he wanted to, he engaged with us, and subsequently, we gained a very clear but complex insight into his illness. If we had taken a more directive approach, the outcome would not have been the same, and would have run the risk of reinforcing core beliefs about the service. After two years of work he is saying that he has a thought disorder and may have schizophrenia.

The reasons that we are generally unable to take this approach with our clients are many, but it may be that it again confronts us with our own inadequacies; we may not want to know the answers so we do not ask the question. It is challenging for us as individuals as well as professionals; it is much harder to work with the client on their level than it is to dictate and prescribe care.

We must therefore look at ourselves. We should be sharing our skills and working together on these very difficult clients, rather than being precious, dismissive, dictatorial and presumptuous.

References

Abdullah SN (1995) Towards individualised clients care implications for education. Journal of Advanced Nursing 22(4): 715.

Allen C (1992) Occupational Therapy Treatment Goals for the Physically and Cognitively Disabled. American Occupational Therapy Association Inc., Bethesda, Md.

Argyle M (1983) Sources of satisfaction and conflict in long-term relationships. Journal of Marriage and the Family 45: 481–493.

Argyle M (1985) The Anatomy of Relationships. Penguin, London.

Barham P (1992) Closing the Asylum: The mental patient in modern society. Penguin, London

Becker H (1970) Sociological Work. Allen Lane, London

Birchwood M, Tarrier N (1994) Psychological Management of Schizophrenia. Wiley, Chichester.

Boyle S, Andrews M (1992) Transcultural Concepts in Nursing Care. Scott, Foresman, Glenview, Ill.

Chadwick P, Birchwood M, Trower P (1996) Cognitive Therapy for Delusions, Voices and Paranoia. Wiley, Chichester.

Chevalier M (1997) Occupational therapy and the search for meaning. Journal of Occupational Therapy 60(12): 539–540.

Crabtree J (1998) The end of occupational therapy. American Journal of Occupational Therapy 52(3): 205–214.

Creek P (1992) Occupational Therapy and Mental Health Principles, Skills and Practice. Churchill Livingstone, Edinburgh.

Day P (1981) Social Work and Social Control. Tavistock, London.

Dingwall R (1977) The Social Organisation of Health Visitor Training. Croom Helm, London.

Ekdawi MY, Conning AM (1994) Psychiatric Rehabilitation: A practice guide. Chapman & Hall, London.

Fair A (1999) Making a cup of tea as part of a culturally sensitive service. British Journal of Occupational Therapy 62(5): 199.

Fowler D, Kuipers L, Garety P (1995) Cognitive Behaviour Therapy for Psychosis. Wiley, Chichester.

Gamble C, Brennan G (2000) Working with Serious Mental Illness. A manual for clinical practice. Baillière Tindall, London.

Garety P, Fowler D, Kuipers L (2000) Cognitive behavioural therapy for medication-resistant symptoms of schizophrenia. Schizophrenia Bulletin 26(1): 73–86.

Hawker R (1989) For the good of the patient? In: Nursing History: The state of the art. Croom Helm, London.

Haywood P, Kemp R, David A (2000) Compliance therapy in psychotic patients: randomised controlled trial. British Medical Journal 312: 345–349.

Hinshelwood RD (1999) The difficult patient. British Journal of Psychiatry 174: 187–190.

Hugman R (1991) Power in Caring Professions. Macmillan, London.

Jahoda M (1981) Work, employment and underemployment. American Psychologist 36: 184–191.

Keddy B, Gillis MJ, Jacobs P, Burton H, Rogers M (1986) The doctor–nurse relationship: an historical perspective. Journal of Advanced Nursing 11(6): 745–753.

Kingdon D, Turkington D (1991) The use of cognitive behaviour therapy with a normalising rationale in schizophrenia. Journal of Nervous and Mental Disorder 179: 207–211.

Macdonald EM (1970) Occupational Therapy in Rehabilitation, 3rd edn. Baillière, Tindall & Cassell, London.

Mayers CA (2000) Casson memorial lecture, Reflect on the past to shape the future. British Journal of Occupational Therapy 63(8): 358.

Meyer A (1977) The philosophy of occupational therapy. American Journal of Occupational Therapy 31: 639.

Mocellin G (1988) A perspective on the principles and practice of occupational therapy. British Journal of Occupational Therapy 51(1): 4–7

Murphy E (1991) After The Asylums: Community Care for People with Mental Illness. Faber and Faber, London.

NICE (2002) Clinical Guidelines: Schizophrenia. Department of Health, London

Ornstein R and Carsten L (1991) Psychology: The Study of Human Experience, 3rd edn. Harcourt Brace Jovanovich, USA

Paloutzian R, Ellison C (1982) Loneliness, spiritual well-being and the quality of life. In: Loneliness. Wiley, New York.

Parsons T (1952) The Social System. Tavistock, London.

Pithouse A (1987) Social Work: The social organisation of an invisible trade. Avebury, Aldershot.

Rathus S, Nevid J (1989) Psychology and the Challenges of Life. Holt, Rinehart, Winston, New York.

Rickman J, Goldthorpe W (1977) When was your last period? In: Health Care and Knowledge, Croom Helm, London.

Ross D (1993) Community care: users' perspectives. In: Dimensions of Community Health Care. Saunders, London.

Satyamurti C (1981) Occupational Survival. Basil Blackwell, Oxford.

Sines B (1994) The arrogance of power: a reflection on contemporary mental health nursing. Journal of Advanced Nursing 20:894–903.

Sullivan P (1994) Recovery from schizophrenia: what we can learn from developing nations. Innovations and Research 3(2).

Trower P, Bryant B, Argyle M (1978) Social Skills and Mental Health. Methuen, London.

Turner JS (1974) Lifespan Development, 3rd edn. Holt, Rinehart and Winston, New York

Turner G, Ten Hoor D (1986) The NINH Community Support Programme: pilot approach to a needed social forum. Community Mental Health Journal 22(1): 4.

Wallis MA (1987) 'Profession' and 'professionalism' and the emerging profession of occupational therapy. British Journal of Occupational Therapy 50(8): 259–262.

Waxler NE (1977) Is mental illness cured in traditional societies. Culture, Medicine, and Psychiatry 1: 233–253.

Wilding P (1982) Professional Power and Social Welfare. Routledge, London.

Williams D, Harrison J et al. (1987) Crafts: a criminal offence? British Journal of Occupational Therapy 50(1): 12–15.

CHAPTER FIVE

Nursing aspects of schizophrenia

SUE KERR

The distress experienced and behaviourally presented by individuals suffering from schizophrenia is frightening, bizarre, at times aggressive and superficially may seem beyond understanding. However, the vernacular of psychiatric nurses is that of a holistic approach to care. The persistent criticisms of psychiatric nursing care suggest a distinctive but intangible quality surrounding, 'knowing everything but choosing what to consider meaningful'. Undoubtedly, the meaningful choice is based on individual knowledge, personal and professional, as well as the social and political constraints of their particular practice environment. However, the code of professional conduct (Nursing and Midwifery Council 2002) outlines key areas of professional practice. These include putting the interests of patients first at all times, the importance of effective teamworking, and respecting patients' rights to confidentiality and their consent to treatment. Moreover, the code sets out an explicit requirement to promote the interests of all patients, in particular the need to acknowledge the special arrangements governing the consent of those detained under the mental health legislation. Psychiatric nurses may need to reappraise their practice in order that these principles are followed.

Schizophrenia is a complex and exquisitely personal experience; the needs of individual sufferers are diverse and distinct, and invariably defy a singular treatment modality. However, as with all distressed beings, a need to understand and work with a meaningful and consistent concept is paramount to collaborative care. The thrust towards an evidence base for health care has to acknowledge various knowledge philosophies. The technical-scientific approach to knowledge imposes a considerable burden on health care by enforcing a science-based technology on medicine in its striving to preserve health (Schon 1987). A 'constructivist' view of knowledge would argue that true knowledge is created in the minds of people, rather than discovered in the outside world (Rolfe et al 2001). Moreover, Schon (1987. p .40) suggested that 'knowing is in the action' which is dynamic, and based on 'facts', 'procedures', 'rules', and 'theories', which are static. This suggests that achieving a collaborative stance requires consideration of numerous experiences and theories. However, the dilemma for health care in particular is that individuals are exactly that – individuals – so to imply one truth for all can be little more than categorical social control. This chapter in particular, and this book as a whole, asks mainly that the reader should think about the rationale for their individual approach to the care of their clients' distress. Science needs to be applied with care and with due consideration for the individual involved. The complex issue of informed consent in the care of schizophrenia has to be considered, given that psychiatry has undeniably an aspect of social control.

Historical overview of psychiatric nursing

If we assume the basic principle of 'care' of being available to offer assistance to those in need, psychiatric nursing existed long before schizophrenia was perceived as an illness. For centuries people in mental distress were herded into 'houses' where they were cared for or contained by individuals who collectively took responsibility for their welfare. Literature cites infirmaries for sick people as early as the tenth century (Cartwright 1977, p. 44). The nature of the sicknesses is ill defined, but the inhabitants of the infirmaries undoubtedly included people suffering some form of mental distress, given the many descriptions of 'Bedlam' in the fifteenth century. In addition, many mentally distressed people were contained in private madhouses, workhouses and prisons. Foucault (1967) describes this time as that of 'great confinement', during which any one who challenged the moral values of the conservative class was considered deviant and separated from society. Many critics of modern psychiatry (Barnham 1984, Szasz 1994) would suggest that society's motivation remains the same in the twenty-first century and that psychiatry is a product of social control.

The late eighteenth century is generally accepted as the era of enlightenment, bringing about a scientific approach along with the beginning of the reform of the inhumane 'madhouses'. Phillipe Pinel (1745–1826) is well known for his reforming work at the Bicêtre in Paris, where he ordered the removal of the chains restraining patients and advocated moral care. Pinel believed that mental illness resulted from a combination of both heredity and life experiences (Kales 1990), a concept that is still under investigation 200 years on.

The doctrine of moral treatment laid the foundations of the therapeutic relationship, advocating support of the dependency needs of the mentally ill. This approach to care was given greater impetus by the onset of King George III's mental illness in 1788. The House of Lords appointed an enquiry into the king's care. The Lunacy Asylum Enabling Act 1808 resulted from this enquiry, suggesting that each county should set up public asylums. However, it took the passing of the Poor Law Amendment Act 1834, which brought the workhouses into being, and consequently highlighted the large numbers of mentally ill housed in them who were unable to work, to bring about the Victorian asylum movement.

The 1845 Lunacy Act forced local authorities to provide accommodation for the mad, and hailed the commissioning of large asylums in every county. Large asylums were built throughout England and Wales, generally away from populated areas. By the end of the nineteenth century, there were 100,000 patients in public asylums (Murphy 1991). The building of the asylums continued, along with the certification of madness, which provided the patients to fill them. The great Victorian asylum era, essentially 'apartheid of the mentally distressed', was established, and reigned for more than 100 years. By 1954, the population of psychiatric institutions reached its peak of 148,000 (Murphy 1991).

The population of England and Wales increased threefold between 1800 and 1900. Detention in asylums, however, increased 20-fold. The disparity between these figures may be indicative of the Victorian attitudes of self-righteousness, and movement from the workhouses to asylums. They may also indicate the lack of clear diagnostic criteria for mental illness.

The asylum movement separated the mentally distressed from other deviant groups, and it also initiated the medicalization and control of those deemed to be mentally disturbed. However, little was understood about the cause of the individual disturbance and even less about any effective treatments. The treatments – most of which were enforced – were based on little more than empirical observations, and would now be considered to breach human rights. Details of these treatments are cited in historical literature; my concern here is to highlight the role of nurses in the procedures.

Throughout this period, men and women were employed to ensure that basic levels of physiological needs were met, and to support and deliver many of the treatments prescribed. These individuals were the precursors of today's mental health nurses. Substantial numbers of mental health nurses still practising were trained in asylums: given an average working life of 40 years, many practising mental health nurses are likely to have participated in this kind of psychiatric care.

The focus of institutional care undoubtedly met the patient's basic physiological needs of shelter, food, and warmth. A large number of institutions were self-sufficient, in that many patients and nurses were employed in maintaining this status. Life in these institutions was rigid, demanding a uniformed passive approach to the daily life of patients and nurses alike.

Release from institutional care was little more than a downsizing of accommodation. The ethos of social care and constraint continued and flourished, mainly due to the media reporting of the failures of community care.

Physical treatments increased from the 1930s onwards, requiring an increased nursing role in medical interventions. This role culminated in the discovery of antipsychotic drugs, prescribed by doctors and administered by nurses. The role of administrating medication continues to be the mainstay of the mental health nurse's daily task.

The historical base of psychiatric nursing has grown from medical constructs of schizophrenia. It is constrained by hierarchies, rules, and the omnipotence of the medical profession (Clarke 1999).

Current status of psychiatric nursing

The concern within this discussion is the submissive compliance with a profession (medicine) which is bound by its inherent biomedical scientific stance and therefore represents an opposing paradigm to that of nursing, which aspires to care from a bio-psychosocial perspective. This compliance bears many similarities to that expected of sufferers from schizophrenia. If nurses' roles are defined by the prescribed treatments of doctors, can they continue to call themselves a professional group when they have no professional power? They are merely agents of medical staff, dispensing medication and reporting changes in mood and behaviour (Carpenter 1989), along with maintaining conformity to a busy schedule of ward activities, and more generally keeping social order in the ward and in the community.

The historical precedent of control of people suffering from schizophrenia has left an indelible mark on psychiatric nurses. A conspiracy of fear is ingrained throughout psychiatric practice. Stories of violent incidents are rife, and regularly repeated. Little attention is given to the success stories, which are numerous by comparison. Generally these stories are dismissed and deemed irrelevant; in fact psychiatry is morbidly bound by its own anxieties of failure, which are often a reflection of public ignorance. The media interest in sensational reporting of homicides, particularly those committed by people suffering from some form of mental distress, has greatly increased professional anxiety.

Medicine in general, and nursing in particular, is also trapped within the opposing dimensions of science. Medicine has the heroic status of curing, extending and improving the quality of life. Psychiatry has taken on the additional task of managing that life within society's rules. Psychiatric nurses act as servants to this role in that they collude with the rules, often as a direct order from other professionals. However, compliance with orders does not negate the responsibility of 'care' that nurses sign up to by accepting their registration.

People with schizophrenia, as well as others in mental distress, live with the daily threat of having their liberty denied, in addition to enforced treatments, at a time when they are most confused and unable to solve problems or explain their dilemma: a time when the concept of care should be to 'nurse' the individual through and back to their everyday life. However, the prevailing view is that people with schizophrenia do not know what's best for them because of their illness. This view is based on a concept of the world that is distinctly 'deluded' in relation to the distress experienced by these individuals. Professional experience colludes with the idea that individuals 'feel' better when they comply with treatment, usually medication. How is the concept of 'feeling better' judged if we don't understand or believe what individual sufferers tell us is true for them? Behavioural presentation is often the yardstick by which 'feeling better' is measured or reported, and provides the empirical evidence that the prescribed treatment is effective.

However, what choice do individuals have but to go along with this charade? The consequence of challenging it is likely to be further coercion, or even being accused of 'abusing' or refusing help that is offered. Evidence (Hirsch and Jolley 1989) suggests that these people are caught in a power struggle with services. Generally, this is met with demands for greater powers to compel individuals to comply (Perkins and Reeper 1998, p. 31). Unfortunately, psychiatric nurses are inextricably bound by these practices, given the very nature of their role to care for these individuals.

The role afforded to psychiatric nurses is bound by their own individual values and the expectations of the institution, which in itself imposes a collective sense of order. The time commitment nurses have to patients is similar to that of sufferers' families: an interesting analogy when one considers the lack of care and consideration accorded to relatives who provide a substantial amount of care and support, with little more than their life experiences to guide them. Additionally, relatives are caught in the emotional turmoil of loss of expectations, guilt and frustration, which are understandably displaced on to a service that fails to meet their family's needs. On reflection, the roles of psychiatric nurses and families are blurred. By definition nursing is akin to the role of parenting, if being available to offer assistance is accepted as a core characteristic of nursing. However, the emotional burden and psychological bonds are intrinsically different, although the potential for transference and countertransference issues is substantially overwhelming, and may be the very essence of professional difficulties. The virulent expression of emotion within psychiatric professions requires investigation in the interests of practitioners and clients. We may need to confront the fact that the frustrations of clients and their families are mirrored by the frustrations of practitioners, who feel similarly uncared for.

The Department of Health document *Working in Partnership* (1994) suggests that mental health nursing should re-examine every aspect of its policy and practice in the light of the needs of the people who use services (p. 5). In addition, it states that nursing interventions should be founded on a sound understanding of the individuals in their care (p. 18).

Nurses are in an excellent position to take up this opportunity, but it demands an alternative emphasis on the therapeutic relationship so often espoused as the focus of psychiatric nursing. The quality of the therapeutic relationship has to take into account the characteristics of the nurse, the client and the situation. These are bound by the reality that we all construct our relationships to meet specific needs. Whether these relationships are positive and or productive will rely on individual and social interpretation.

The crux of this for psychiatric nurses will be their ability to acknowledge and understand personal and social interpretations from the perspective of a person with schizophrenia. This is potentially a personal journey of discovery for the sufferer and the nurse. However, a departure from history, its anxieties and empirical evidence, is necessary if nurses are to embrace collaborative working with schizophrenia, and other carers. Morrall's (1998, p. 43) study of psychiatric nursing and social control asks whether psychiatric nurses have control over their clinical practice. The conclusion suggests that the domination of psychiatric nursing by psychiatry results in the former being tied to the social control function of the latter. Moreover, psychiatric nurses are caught within a schizophrenic analogy of opposing dimensions of 'care and control'. However, this may be a double bind of our own making, considering the incessant objections made by nurses to the medical model, while we continuing to comply with its demands, under the disguise of medical dominance. Morrall (1998), Barker (1999), Clarke (1999) and many others see the real focus of psychiatric nursing as one of social change by the use of a productive therapeutic relationship based on the real needs of individual sufferers: a relationship that enables these individuals to truly live within the community, a collaboration that lives up to its definition of working together against the enemy. The enemy must be the distress and social stigma experienced by people with schizophrenia, not the other professionals engaged in the fight.

Functional analysis of psychiatric nursing

A functional analysis requires a descriptive account of the subject under study. By its very nature, it tends to be based on the behaviour of the subject within any given situation. Therefore, it offers the opportunity to explicate the basics of a collaborative approach to psychiatric care.

Schizophrenia for both the sufferer and the world around them is embedded in fear – of the unknown, the inexplicable – and misunderstanding; a description of most people's nightmares at their worst. The analogy of dreaming while awake is often used to describe schizophrenia, but is at best only an apology for the real distress of the experience. Historically, these experiences were defined as a product of illness, so any attempts to understand them within the context of the lived experience were deemed to be useless and perhaps even an exacerbating factor (Scharfetter 1980). Therefore, sufferers were left to seek their own understanding of personally 'real' experiences that often continued despite treatment. It is hardly surprising that many of these individuals formulated intricate and creative rationales for their experiences. The rationales were beyond 'normal' understanding; however, the experiences themselves generally failed to fit with normal experience. Therefore they remained inexplicable, though the opportunity to discuss the experiences within the normal dimension of experiences would go some way to understanding the intricate rationales. Providing a framework, however tentative, on which individuals can base an understanding of the confusing and frightening experience of schizophrenia would seem likely to provide reassurance, reduce anxiety, and ease feelings of depression; in others words, talking about the experience may have a direct therapeutic potential (Kingdom and Turkingdon 1994). Therefore, nurses need to engage with sufferers and their families in collaboration against the fear instilled through the experiences.

Given that we still lack an effective primary prevention of schizophrenia, nurses need to make great efforts to improve our secondary knowledge. As long as this disorder persists as one of our most costly medical conditions, economically as well as in terms of human suffering, any clinically significant reduction in the severity or duration of acute schizophrenia is surely worth the investment (Vaglum 1996). Psychiatric nurses are in the optimum position to meet this challenge. People with schizophrenia are in need of steady and clear human relationships, calm and benevolent attitudes, 'talking and togetherness' (Watson 1990). This process may help to reduce the individual's emotional distress by the process of containing their feelings and being receptive to their experience, being able to bear and think constructively about these feelings (Bowles et al. 2002).

This identifies 'what' nurses need to do – listen, acknowledge, and attempt to understand the 'fear' of the experience. However, this may be the very nature of the problem. Nurses, like all other health care professionals, are a diverse collection of individuals, all with their own interpretation of themselves, the world and others. This provides a wealth of opportunities as well as some distressing experiences. An individual's ability to cope with the intense anxiety and pain associated with mental distress will vary considerably. Nurse education, practice development and clinical supervision often fail to recognize the individual needs of nurses – a replication of the process that sufferers experience with psychiatry. Therefore, nurses are often fraught with anxiety in relation to their own psychological safety. This anxiety is often displaced on to patients and colleagues, unfortunately bound within a passive-aggressive and hostile presentation.

Nurses reading this may feel heavily criticized, even insulted at this point, and they deserve an explanation. The reality is that most psychiatric nurses care deeply about their patients and seek to ensure their safety. However, the concept of safety is seriously distorted by a lack of individualized understanding. An environment that is safe, supportive, tolerant and accepting is generally one that we all desire. Individuals with schizophrenia are no different. Environments are rarely consistently stable all the time, but psychiatric nurses need to engender this stability if they are to meet the specific needs of those with schizophrenia and their patients in general. Failing to ensure this need amounts to little more than neglect.

However, the remit of acute psychiatric care in particular has extended beyond the care of schizophrenia and other clearly defined mental illnesses. Acute wards have become intensive care units, expected to provide care for severely disturbed individuals, many afflicted with complex and distressing personality traits as well as mental disorders. Student psychiatric nurses and newly qualified nurses work for substantial periods on these units: in fact this experience is seen as the front line of psychiatry, the apprenticeship of a psychiatric nurse. This could in fact be true if the focus was on 'care' rather than 'control'. Undoubtedly, there is a need for control of the distress experienced by individuals. However, the enviable context in which nurses find themselves is that of working with patients 24 hours a day. This must be a unique opportunity to understand the difficulty individuals have with their lives: an opportunity to compare and contrast what relieves an individual's distress, what helps them to achieve personal care, an opportunity to explore the antecedents that led to the need for intensive care. Given the confusion people with schizophrenia experience in their relationships with others, this requires predictable responses, which are explained and based on a rational process. Variable, inconsistent and unpredictable responses are generally disagreeable to us all; to someone with schizophrenia they are a cause of substantial stress. A normal expectation of any interactions is clarity – explaining any unexpected changes and acknowledging the distress and frustration this may cause. Moreover, the validity of an individual's opinions and beliefs should be acknowledged as important for them, not merely delusional or psychotic. People with schizophrenia are invariably hypersensitive and often feel overwhelmed by excessive or confusing stimulation and in need of clear and concise communication, which is paced at a level acceptable to the individual. They need time to clarify and explain understanding, and acceptance is likely to reduce misunderstanding for both parties.

Although people with schizophrenia need everyone's support and encouragement in abundance, they also have rights and responsibilities as members of society. Psychiatric nurses, unfortunately, are often in the unenviable position of reinforcing these social responsibilities. Martindale (2001, p. 29) exposes the continuing lack of attention to, and use of, existing and available knowledge, particularly of the mental processes that take place between patients and groups of staff at different organizational levels. This failure accounts for much of our present inability to provide consistent, quality services and care for people with schizophrenia. However, exploring the antecedents to any given behaviour requires an understanding of the motivations that drive that particular behaviour. Motivation is a complex, multidimensional and integrated process, and beyond the remit of this chapter. Moreover, it detracts from the essence of what is being discussed – psychosis and the personality traits of the individual sufferer and possibly those of the people interacting with them.

'State' versus 'trait'

Grotstein (2001, p. 10) discusses the concept of 'state' versus 'trait', highlighting the normality of personality traits, in that they are what constitutes our psychic individuality. However, these traits have the potential to precipitate, maintain or exacerbate a psychotic state. This does not negate the known physiological factors that precipitate psychosis; they are additional factors, and relevant to the therapeutic approach to schizophrenia. The nursing care of people with schizophrenia has been confused by the emergence of the borderline condition as a diagnostic entity, in that this has provided psychiatric nurses with a tangible explanation or excuse for the difficulties they experience with many patients. Undoubtedly, this problem is not unique to nurses, and collectively may constitute a large part of the failings for which the mental health services are criticised.

Within therapeutic relationships considerable emphasis is placed on compliance with any given intervention. It is true to say that a therapeutic alliance with someone who has a borderline personality trait requires specific and consistent skills, which are not generally taught to or practised by psychiatric nurses. Therefore, the displaced anxiety engendered by this trait in particular, and others generally, inevitably leads to it being used as the scapegoat for many and varied difficulties within psychiatric nursing. This does not negate the real service issues for this group of distressed individuals. What is important is the impact the lack of clarity about these individuals' needs has on people with schizophrenia and how their psychotic difficulties are misunderstood as personality trait difficulties. Therefore, the ensuing conundrum is that personality traits have an important bearing on an individual psychosis and need to be acknowledged within the treatment profile.

Grotstein (2001, p. 10) further reminds us that antipsychotic medications, like all psychotropic agents, affect state disorders such as psychosis, but no medication affects trait disorders, which periodically or permanently sub-tend the psychosis. This must pose an ethical question in relation to the use of psychotropic medication in managing behaviour which may not be driven by a psychosis. Services have a responsibility to debate this issue and nurses have the obligation to justify their part in such a process, given the conse-quences in relation to their professional code of conduct.

Support for mental health workers

Hinshelwood (1999) highlights the personal cost of working with psychosis (states) and/or personality disorders (traits) and the subtle game played by professionals of shifting from one diagnosis to the other in order to manage our own anxiety. Martindale (2001, p. 28) expands on this suggestion by highlighting that mental health professionals have learned that working with the seriously emotionally disturbed is itself highly disturbing (though they have not learned from the experience). Being in the presence of psy-chosis sooner or later generates extreme thoughts and feelings in all of us, which can be deeply unsettling. If mental health workers generally, and psy-chiatric nurses in particular, are to manage this disturbance on a daily basis they will need considerable emotional support themselves: a luxury which most services neither have nor advocate. Many mental health services are struggling to ensure all health workers receive a basic level of clinical super-vision, though this in itself may be another anxiety reduction process, given the increased demand for risk assessment. Therefore, psychiatric nurses, particularly ward-based staff, have little choice but to displace and avoid their own anxiety. The consequences of this process are social control of individual sufferers and control of psychiatry's anxieties. A primitive but effective survival plan.

Regaining values: the collaborative approach

What are psychiatric nurses to do in order to regain the values that brought them into a caring profession? Kelly and Field (1994) state that the psychi-atric profession argues that the only value its members promote is health, and claim that professional neutrality with respect to all other values relieves them of the need to consider ethics in the philosophical sense. Moreover, Kelly and Field argue that this position may, unconsciously, introduce a wide range of personal, social or political values into clinical practice, conse-quently highlighting the need for a collaborative approach that is based on individual needs and the collective evidence for the proposed intervention. Nurses are generally on the front line of this care proposal, in that they spend considerably more time with clients than any other professional. The opportunity to identify and present an individual profile of the client's needs is unique to the nursing profession. However, we need to encompass the values of individuality, rationality and balance (Michaels 1994). Additionally, Kelly and Field (1994) suggest curiosity, relatedness and responsibility. Reflection on these values require individual practitioners to explore the meaning of everyday value statements made about clients, the most pertinent being the use of 'appropriate' as a definition of an individual's behaviour. Would you be able to apply this term collectively to your colleagues? Would they apply it to you (food for thought)?

The model of nursing proposed by Barker and Walker (2000) is colloquially known as the 'tidal' model, given its proposition that individuals' mental health needs ebb and flow as does the tide. It further suggests the need to collaborate with others, including clients, to provide what is needed when it is needed. Resources are scarce, so a finely tuned consistent approach with clear and shared aims which are specific to the individual's needs can be cost-effective as well as productive for all involved. The criticisms aimed at psychiatry generally suggest that this approach is rare. Those aimed at nurses are specifically focused on the lack of therapeutic alliance between nurses and their clients. In order for this situation to be rectified, everyone involved in the education, practice and management of psychiatry may need to explore the values they currently hold in relation to their application of their practice. Kelly and Field (1994) propose that psychiatry should be governed by the virtue of 'humility', which would allow us to appreciate the limits of our ability to understand and influence others' experiences, and recognize the narrowness of our expertise and the danger of claiming authority beyond it. Moreover, it may enable psychiatric nurses to acknowledge the unique position they employ within psychiatry and their client's lives: that of co-operation, convergence and divergence of approaches based on the unique ability to understand individual client's needs, given time and freedom from any treatment belief that lacks an appropriate clinical rationale. Nurses have the opportunity to be the client's consultant on the best available treatment approaches; however, they need to ensure that this opportunity is supported by their own knowledge base and acknowledge personal and professional limitations.

Co-operation could support the growth of a climate wherein new learning develops through rational dialogue and constructive assessment of the merits and limitations of collaborative work (Jackson, 2001). Moreover, Jackson proposes that

> to change polarized attitudes and reduce poor-quality work clinicians (nurses) must, as Michael Balint recommended, work together to distinguish, in each case, between what we can do, what we might do had we the resources, what we must do, and what we are under the circumstances, going to do.

All these improvements begin with individual health care workers. Moreover, psychiatric nurses need to explore the rationale for their own dissatisfaction with their practice, and look to the changes they can personally make in collaboration with all involved in individual cases of care.

Educational requirements

Nurses have been introduced to a wide and variable range of biological, psychological and social theories of the causation and treatment of mental distress. However, the concerns and criticisms continue, as do the inter-professional disagreements about the real focus of nursing. Psychiatric nurse education has undergone numerous curriculum changes in the past 30 years, in terms of academic perspective, theoretical focus and skills base. Training for mental health nurses was the responsibility of health authorities until the introduction of Project 2000 in the mid-1980s moved nurse education into the higher education framework, in addition to a curriculum that delivered a 'common foundation programme' to all nurses for the first half of their training. This was seen as demoting psychiatric nursing to a post-basic speciality (Dingwall et al. 1988).

Psychiatric nurses are caught in an educational and organizational conflict of opposing paradigms of care. Morral (1998) suggests that psychiatric nursing in Britain is confronted by a multitude of external determinants. They include:

- the prolonged period of fiscal restraint, inaugurated by a succession of Conservative governments (likely to continue under the present Labour government), which has meant a significant reduction in state expenditure on public services
- the possibility of a reversal of the policy of decarcerating the mentally ill in the light of unabated criticism of care in the community
- the production of yet more official reports attempting to clarify the role of the psychiatric nurse.

Surely the question has to be 'Why is psychiatric nursing so difficult to define'? Moreover, if we don't know what it is, what do we educate psychiatric nurses to do?

Or is the question how to be? The innovative work of Menzies (1960) highlighted the impact of the patient's suffering on nurses, and that much of nurses' work was designed in such a way as to protect them from significant emotional contact. Moreover, the strain of attempting to integrate biological, psychological and social approaches to individuals' care can lead to splitting processes by staff, leading to a polarization of thinking amongst the staff group and to idealization of the easier forms of therapy with denigration of others (Martindale 2001, p. 31).

This phenomenon is not limited to psychoanalytical interpretations: similar outcomes have been replicated in the numerous evaluations of family work for schizophrenia (Leff et al. 1990). Considerable evidence exists to support the validity and efficacy of working with these families. Moreover, it is work that can be readily taught to psychiatric nurses. However, the reality is that very few families receive this support. Therefore, mere knowledge and skills apparently fail to provide competent and confident psychiatric nurses. A fundamental aspect of nurse education may be missing: that of the nature and burden of care. Although a sound knowledge base is a requisite for psychiatric care, the increasing demand for evidence-based care may have a detrimental effect on the psychiatric nurse's ability to hold on to the (painful) knowledge of working with individuals with psychoses, which will, by its very nature, always lead to a vulnerability to distortion of interpersonal processes affecting staff and their organizations, (Martindale 2001). Therefore, nurse educators need to explore techniques that enable psychiatric nurses to understand, hold and defuse the painful experiences of working with people who are mentally ill. This requires a consistent approach from all those involved, in addition to the ability to work collaboratively.

The approach one engenders may have less of a therapeutic outcome than the ability to provide consistent and clear approaches to care. An approach to education that provides overviews of numerous theories, without any attempt to enable psychiatric nurses to conceptualize the theories to understanding human suffering, negates the concept of holistic care, which by its nature requires considerable knowledge and skills to be able to sensitively explore and meet all of an individual's needs. Therefore, a return to the basic, though fundamental concept of 'care' as a notion of 'being with' the individual experiencing mental distress and providing some containment for the consequential emotional pain may be the very essence of psychiatric nursing: a quality and skill that requires enormous compassion for the individual sufferer, an ability to rationalize and balance the interpersonal process experienced in each and every relationship. It also requires an evolving curiosity in relation to the knowledge and skills of others, and the ability to take responsibility for advocating a collaboration of approaches, based on an in-depth knowledge of individual difficulties and the skill of conceptualizing the interrelation of individual thoughts, feelings and behaviour given the environment in which they currently exist.

However, such an elegant and essentially simple approach requires the acknowledgement and respect of psychiatric nurses themselves. The integrity of psychiatric nursing has to be underpinned by a belief in the need for everyday compassion to relieve human distress, while acknowledging the limitations of our own values and beliefs.

References

Barker P (1999) The Philosophy and Practice of Psychiatric Nursing. Churchill Livingstone, London.

Barker P and Walker L (2000) Nurses' perceptions of multidisciplinary teamwork in acute psychiatric settings. Journal of Psychiatric and Mental Health Nursing 7(6): 539.

Barnham P (1984) Schizophrenia and Human Values. Blackwell, Oxford.

Bowles N, Dodds P, Hackney D, Sunderland C, Thomas P (2002) Formal Observations and engagement: a discussion paper. Journal of Psychiatric and Mental Health Nursing 9: 255–260.

Carpenter M (1989) Asylum nursing, A chapter in the history of labour. In Davies C (ed) Re-writing Nursing History, Croom Helm, Hampshire.

Cartwright FF (1977) A Social History of Medicine. Longman, London.

Clarke L (1999) Challenging Ideas in Psychiatric Nursing. Routledge, London.

Department of Health (1994) Working in Partnership: A Collaborative Approach To Care. HMSO, London.

Dingwall R, Rafferty AM, Webster C (1988) An Introduction to the Social History of Nursing. Routledge, London.

Foucault M (1967) Civilisation – A History of Insanity in the Age of Reason. Tavistock, London.

Grotstein JS (2001) A rationale for the psychoanalytically informed psychotherapy of schizophrenia and other psychoses: towards the concept of 'rehabilitative psychoanalysis'. Chapter 1 in Williams P (ed.), A Language for Psychosis. Whurr Publishers, London.

Hinshelwood RD (1999) The difficult patient. British Journal of Psychiatry 174: 187–190.

Hirsch SR, Jolley AG (1989) The dysphoric syndrome of schizophrenia and its implications for relapse. British Journal of Psychiatry 156: 46–50.

Jackson M (2001) Psychoanalysis and the treatment of psychosis. Chapter 3 in Williams P (ed.), A Language for Psychosis. Whurr Publishers, London.

Kales A, Kales JD, Vela-Bueno A (1990) Schizophrenia: Historical Perspectives. In Kales A, Stephanis C and Talbot I (eds), Recent Advances in Schizophrenia. Springer Verlag, New York.

Kelly MP, Field D (1994) Comments on the rejection of the biomedical model in sociological discourse. Medical Sociological News 19(2): 34–37.

Kingdom D, Turkingdon D (1994) Cognitive-behavioural Interventions in Psychotic Disorders. Routledge, London.

Leff J, Berkowitz R, Shavit N, Strachan A, Glass I, Vaughn C (1990) A trial of family therapy versus a relatives group for schizophrenia, a two year follow-up. British Journal of Psychiatry 157: 571–577.

Martindale B (2001) New discoveries concerning psychoses and their organisational fate. Chapter 2 in Williams P (ed.), A Language for Psychosis. Whurr Publishers, London.

Menzies I (1960) A case study in the functioning of social systems as a defence against anxiety. Human Relations 13: 95–121.

Michaels S (1994) Invisible skills: how recognition and value need to be given to the 'invisible skills' frequently used by mental health nurses, but often unrecognised by those familiar with mental health nursing. Journal of Psychiatric and Mental Health Nursing 1(1): 56–57.

Morrall P (1998) Mental Health Nursing and Social Control. Whurr Publishers, London.

Murphy E (1991) After the Asylums. Faber & Faber, London

Nursing and Midwifery Council (2002) Professional Code of Conduct. The Stationery Office, London.

Perkins RE, Repper J (1998) Principles of working with people who experience mental health problems. Chapter 2 in Brokker C, Repper J (eds) Serious Mental Health Problems in the Community. Baillière Tindall, London.

Rolfe G, Freshwater D, Jasper M (2001) Critical Reflection for Nursing. Palgrave, Basingstoke.

Scharfetter C (1980) General Psychopathology. Cambridge University Press, Cambridge.

Schon D (1987) Educating the Reflective Practitioner. Jossey-Bass, San Francisco.

Szasz T (1994) Cruel Compassion. Syracuse University Press, New York.

Vaglum P (1996) Early detection in schizophrenia: Unsolved questions. Schizophrenia Bulletin 22(2): 347–351.

Watson R (1990) Accountability in Nursing Practice. Chapman & Hall, London.

Index